BREAST-FEEDING
and the
FOURTH TRIMESTER

BREAST-FEEDING

and the

FOURTH TRIMESTER

A supportive, expert guide
to the first three months

LUCY WEBBER, IBCLC

First published in 2023 by Headline Home
an imprint of Headline Publishing Group

5

Cataloguing in Publication Data is available from the British Library

Trade paperback ISBN 978 1035 40443 8
eISBN 978 1035 40444 5

Typeset in Dante MT by Avon DataSet Ltd, Alcester, Warwickshire

Printed and bound in Great Britain by Clays Ltd, Elcograf S.p.A.

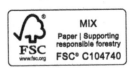

MIX
Paper | Supporting
responsible forestry
FSC® C104740

Headline's policy is to use papers that are natural, renewable and recyclable products
and made from wood grown in well-managed forests and other controlled sources.
The logging and manufacturing processes are expected to conform to the
environmental regulations of the country of origin.

HEADLINE PUBLISHING GROUP
An Hachette UK Company
Carmelite House
50 Victoria Embankment
London EC4Y 0DZ

The authorised representative in the EEA is Hachette Ireland, 8 Castlecourt
Centre, Dublin 15, D15 XTP3, Ireland (email: info@hbgi.ie)

www.headline.co.uk
www.hachette.co.uk

I'd like to dedicate this book to my own babies.
All three have taught me so very much, not least that it's
OK to not know, and it's OK to ask for help.

Without them I wouldn't have been able to work in this
world, support the families I do, or write this book.

Contents

1

The fourth trimester, breastfeeding, and this book

Four trimesters? Aren't there only three?

Don't worry, you're not going to be pregnant for an extra three months! The phrase 'fourth trimester' refers to the first three months of a baby's life *after* they've been born. It's a wonderful whirlwind of a time. Magical, but messy. Terrific, but testing. Surprising, soul affirming and . . . yes, perhaps a little unsettling at times. But you're going to do just great.

When you think about other mammals, they're born pretty self-sufficient, aren't they? Up and walking within minutes, often learning to hunt within weeks. But human babies? Well, they are completely dependent on us – apart from some incredible reflexes – and remain so for a pretty long time.

We often assume birth is when our babies start to become independent, but, in actual fact, it's much slower, a gradual process. Many now call this period the 'fourth trimester', because it can feel like we're creating a continued womb-like environment for them over those first few months. Think of it as extending pregnancy a little longer on the outside, perhaps. Carrying and cradling them, keeping them snug and warm and fed. Letting them grow and develop just that little bit longer before they're ready to start ever so gradually making their own way in the world. Around the 3-to-4-month mark is commonly when a lot of parents feel their baby is starting to show more signs of this; beginning to reach for things, or starting to roll over. They still need you for a lot longer, of course, but, for some, the signs that more independence is beginning are starting to show.

For a lot of you, this fourth trimester will be your introduction to parenthood. For your baby, it's their introduction to their whole life. The love and care you give them now form the building blocks of who they will become. Oof, does that feel like pressure?! There's no need to feel stressed, as you're going to be amazing at this, I promise. But that's why the theme of this book is not just breastfeeding, it's breastfeeding *and* the fourth trimester. Because our expectations of what it will be like often turn out to be a bit out of whack with how it actually is. And society has weird ideas about what we should be doing, what's right and wrong, and, to top it off, we put a lot of unnecessary pressure on ourselves at this time. With this book, I wanted to try to help you break through the noise, and relax into the fourth trimester in a realistic but supported way.

Breastfeeding

I'm going to assume that, by choosing this book, you've chosen to breastfeed, and that's awesome! Great choice.

At this point, I think most people are well aware that breastfeeding and breastmilk are the optimal choice for health for both you and your baby, so I'm not going to bang on too much about that. It can be incredibly unhelpful to keep hearing messages about how important breastfeeding is but then not be supported to do it. What *is* helpful, though, is knowledge, empowerment and support to allow you to breastfeed until you choose to stop, whenever that may be – after one day, one month, one year, or beyond. Every feed is beneficial and should be celebrated.

There are a lot of books about breastfeeding out there, among them some truly fantastic ones,* but what I wanted to give you with *this* book, is a realistic guide to the things you may come across while breastfeeding in the early months, the good and the not quite so good, and help you navigate them to reach *your* goals.

There are certain topics that come up again and again at breast-feeding groups, online forums, and in consultations with lactation consultants like myself. The messages about them can be mixed, or conflicting, and it can all be a bit confusing, so this book is about trying to help you figure it out.

What I hope to achieve above all by writing this book, is to ensure you feel able to reach out for support. To know that you're not alone. And to deeply ingrain a message that you are wonderful, your feelings are valid, and you're doing a *fantastic* job.

What I wish I'd known about the fourth trimester

Here are some things that parents tell me they wish they'd known about the fourth trimester:

'That all my baby actually needed was me.'

'That babies just want to be held. It's 100% normal and you aren't causing problems by doing it.'

---

* At the back of this book you'll find suggestions for further reading. For those of you that want to know more about why breastfeeding is worth doing, please check it out.

'That you don't need to rush to get out and about. Stay in bed/on the sofa for as long as you want to.'

'An emotional rollercoaster. I never knew I could be so hard on myself.'

'That actually I would enjoy every bit!'

'That it really feels like it will last for ever, but it doesn't.'

'How lonely it can be. I wish I'd taken the advice to go to a support group.'

'You don't have to enjoy it. It's okay to find it hard.'

'Frequent feeding is often normal. It worried me so much at the time but now I'd do anything to go back to sitting there feeding and watching Netflix all day!'

'You need to surrender to it, and let go of all your expectations.'

'Embrace the beautiful chaos.'

'I thought it would be really hard, but because I knew to just go with it, I actually really enjoyed it.'

'That babies don't just feed for hunger!'

'That you cannot spoil a baby. You can't give them too much love or cuddles, no matter what.'

'That it's okay to find it hard, and that it's worth every second.'

'It's more important to focus on feeding than getting out and about. There's too much pressure to enjoy maternity leave.'

'GET. A. SLING!'

'That breastfeeding may be natural, but you have to work hard at it to get it going.'

'That it can take time for the love to come, and that's normal.'

'That you'll feel like you've got your tits out 24/7 for weeks.'

'No, you don't need to put them down. Yes, they can be hungry again.'

'It can be so up and down. Easy one day and impossible the next.'

'That you *won't* know what their cries mean!'

'Hormones kick you in the butt.'

'Never craved chocolate so much in my life.'

'You don't need to worry about how you look. The most important thing right now is getting to know your baby and holding them close.'

'It's okay to need a break and not want to always be holding your baby. You're not a bad parent.'

'That breastfeeding support is mixed. That IBCLCs exist!'

Who's who in the world of breastfeeding?

On a practical note, in the UK there are a lot of people you might come across who could support you with breastfeeding. I thought it would be useful to describe who they are right at the start, so you know who's who and consider who might be the best fit so that you can get the best support for you.

Midwife: You'll see a midwife through your pregnancy, birth, and for two to four weeks after your baby arrives. Most NHS Trusts offer their midwives breastfeeding training, though how much they do may vary. For some it may be just a few hours as part of their ongoing training, while others may spend several days going into it in more detail, with yearly updates.

NHS Trusts that have adopted the UNICEF Baby Friendly Initiative are likely to have had more training, however, and have standards they have to adhere to.

'I love to see women develop their skill and confidence with breastfeeding and believe in their own body's ability to feed their baby.' – Belinda, Midwife

Health visitor: Health visitors work with your family from around two weeks after your baby is born up until school age.

Health visitors are qualified nurses or midwives who do a further year of training in public health. They may have been adult nurses, mental health nurses, district nurses, children's nurses or any other type of nurse before getting into health visiting, and this means they have a fantastic collective knowledge of health services, but that, individually, their breastfeeding expertise can vary.

Again, UNICEF Baby Friendly Initiative have standards for community staff that some areas will have adopted.

'For me, breastfeeding support is the most rewarding aspect of the health visitor role. Infant feeding is beautifully *intertwined with early relationship building. So, empowering women to master their own practical and intuitive breast-feeding skills, whilst boosting health and well-being outcomes for themselves and their babies, is wonderful. My best days at work are when I marvel at the strength and determination of mums overcoming breastfeeding challenges, when I share the joy of a mum bursting with happiness at her own success or when I observe a family unit bathing in the glory of all that lovely oxytocin that I helped create through the privilege of uplifting them for a short while.'* – Karen, health visitor

GP/Paediatrician: Doctors' training in breastfeeding in the UK is often optional, and a lot of doctors have done no training in breastfeeding at all.

That said, there are national guidelines they can follow if they're working with someone who is breastfeeding, and they should be able to signpost you to people who are more qualified if they are not.

'I'm proud to be a doctor that supports breastfeeding, and being a consultant paediatrician does put me in a position where I can influence the next and upcoming group of paediatricians and general practitioners.

I am keen to encourage breastfeeding and consciously make a point of remarking positively to parents, no matter where in their journey they are. There are always benefits to breastfeeding, whether it's the best nutrition available, its immunity boosting properties for those babies unlucky enough to be in hospital with bronchiolitis or even more serious illnesses or the ability to give comfort during a procedure such as a heel prick or blood test. There's ways of getting breastmilk to babies even when they are very poorly.' – Phil, Consultant paediatrician.

Peer supporter: You're most likely to find peer supporters at breastfeeding support groups and their attached online forums. They are usually parents who have breastfed themselves and have gone on and done some training to be able to support others. Their training has usually taken between 16 and 36 hours, and they tend to work in voluntary roles.

Their main role is to listen and support, but they can also help you identify if something isn't going well and signpost you to the appropriate people to help.

'I became a breastfeeding peer supporter so that I could support families to achieve their feeding goals in a way that they wanted to. Providing evidence-based information and being able to relate to many problems that families can face (from personal experience) allows peer supporters to offer support in a way that is unique, and person centred.' – Faye, peer supporter.

Breastfeeding counsellor: Breastfeeding counsellors have usually fed their own baby for 6-to-12 months, and have gone on and done up to two years of part time but very in-depth study. They have a lot of knowledge and excellent counselling skills.

You can find them working in a variety of places, from support groups, helplines, online forums, and some work in the NHS.

'It is a great privilege to be supporting breastfeeding families. As a BFC, I've been supporting (mainly) women to give their breastmilk to their babies for over twenty years. I've a real passion for sharing my knowledge (or 'banging on about it', according to my kids). I'm endlessly fascinated by the science and magic of breastmilk and breastfeeding.

The breastfeeding relationship is a precious and important one, one which is often undermined and undervalued. It's way more than just giving milk to an infant. It's empowering a mother to mother in a way that she feels confident.' – Ann, breastfeeding counsellor.

International board certified lactation consultant (IBCLC): The training that IBCLCs undergo is the only internationally recognised breastfeeding qualification. Often described as the gold standard of breastfeeding support, they're the most highly qualified professional. They will have done an extensive background in health sciences, at least 95 hours in lactation-specific education, with at least 1,000 supervised hours of clinical support, and then had to sit rigorous examinations where a minimum score of around 80 per cent is required in order to pass. They must also continually update their education, and recertify every five years to continue to hold this qualification.

You'll find IBCLCs working in a variety of roles, from writing policies and guidelines, implementing the UNICEF BFI standards, training midwives, or running specialist clinics. They cover a wide variety of roles. IBCLCs may work voluntarily or in the NHS, while some are in private practice.

'I love being an IBCLC, because when you are able to understand and solve breastfeeding problems, you can offer families breastfeeding solutions. The people I'm helping can then make choices to feed in a way that feels right to them without grief and pain.' – Josie, IBCLC.

Infant feeding team: Most NHS Trusts have an infant feeding team. These will be the specialists that you'll see if you have any difficulties that are out of the scope of those you would normally see. They may be midwives, health visitors, or, in some places, IBCLCs. Some have a tongue-tie assessment service too. You can get a referral to see them from your midwife, health visitor or GP.

Me! The author of this book: My name is Lucy Webber. I trained in midwifery in the UK after leaving school at eighteen, and have now been a Registered Midwife for over twenty years.

I had my first two babies a few years after I qualified, and was shocked to realise I *really* didn't know much about breastfeeding. I ended up reading, and reading, and reading some more. I became quite the geek about it all! And when a job came up to be an infant-feeding specialist midwife, I jumped at the chance.

Doing that role led me to do loads of additional training around infant feeding (though it still barely scratched the surface) and so I was able to sit my exams and become an International Board Certified Lactation Consultant in 2012.

Between 2011 and 2016, I led the hospital Trust I was working for through the UNICEF Baby Friendly

Accreditation from start to completion, started and ran a tongue-tie division service, and then a specialist clinic for complex breastfeeding problems.

I then had my third baby in 2016, and, for a multitude of reasons, I didn't go back to the NHS, but decided to be a mum for a while. After a bit, I considered getting a job in a café, or my local supermarket, but in my heart I *knew* I couldn't move away from supporting families. I'd worked so hard to get my internationally recognised, and fairly rare, qualification, and it seemed such a shame to waste it. So I decided to potter about doing a little private work and see what happened.

I'm now five years down the line with private practice, and, *my word*, I've learned so much. Staying in contact with so many of these families long term has shown me a huge amount about the realities and practicalities of feeding and parenting a new baby.

I started a Facebook and Instagram page a few years ago, mainly just to let people know I was around for support if needed, but quickly realised there was a lack of articles about things I wanted to share, so I started to write them myself. These articles get widely shared, and seem to resonate so much with parents, which is what led to the birth of this book. I think, and I really do hope, that I've worked out what families need to know and hear, and, rather selfishly, I really enjoy giving families this information and seeing how validated and reassured they feel.

So that's me. That's why you're reading this. I hope it helps. x

2

The first few days with your new baby

Congratulations, they've arrived! . . . what the heck happens now?

If you're anything like me, you will have spent plenty of time thinking about the birth of your baby and not really spared much of a thought to afterwards. Don't worry, you're not alone! And it's going to be okay.

In this chapter we'll have a look at some of the things that may go on in those first few days. There's a real variety of experiences, of course, depending on how many weeks you are when your baby arrives, how much they weigh, how they were born, and lots more. But I'll outline some of the basics so you've got a good idea of what's likely to go on.

Whatever happens, remember they're *your* baby, and you're entitled to all the information to help you make decisions about what happens and when. You're the boss here!

It's really common to feel completely out of your depth, and like you're flailing around a bit. You're not, I promise. You're doing great, just take it one step at a time.

If you have any questions at all, speak to your midwife or health care provider, who can help guide you through your own individual situation.

But, first things first . . .

Skin to skin

As soon as possible after your baby is born, you'll be encouraged to hold them next to your naked chest, no matter how they've been born.

Top tip: if you're squeamish, you can have them dried off first, but please don't worry either way. When it comes to it, you'll actually just want them on you as soon as you can, even if they do resemble a rather slimy jelly baby!

Not only does this skin-to-skin contact help them to regulate their breathing, heart rate and keep them warm, but these cuddles make a big difference to feeding too. These amazing snuggles give your baby a sense of closeness and access to feeds – I mean, let's face it: they're much more likely to look for a feed if they're next to your boob than if they're wrapped up and lying in a cot! Skin to skin helps ramp up your hormones too, and, frankly, the cuddles are just SO nice. You'll be able to really start to get to know your brand new baby and look at that little face you've been waiting to see for so very long.

Do try and spend as much time skin to skin with them in those first few days and weeks as you can, as it's not just for immediately after birth; it's helpful the entire time you're feeding – and beyond. What many don't realise is that every time we kiss and cuddle our babies, we share our healthy microorganisms with them too. It's not just about love, bonding and feeding, you see. It's good for their health too!

The Golden Hour?

So, look, you may have heard about 'the golden hour' (i.e. spending the first hour after birth in uninterrupted skin-to-skin contact). The thing is, circumstances get in the way and sometimes it's just not possible. I'm really sorry if this happens to you, as I know it can be really drummed into you that it's important.

But, while it's undoubtedly a great thing to do if you can, if you *can't* – just try to do it as soon as you *are* able. Whether that's an hour later, or several days later or more. It will still be hugely valuable, it's never too late.

Your first feed

It can vary, but you may find that your first feed will occur during some early skin-to-skin time shortly after birth. What can sometimes happen is that your baby may do what's known as 'the breast crawl'. Babies are born with reflexes and instincts to search for and latch on to the breast, and will often 'crawl' their way over to find it, amazing as that sounds. For healthy babies (and if you're feeling up to it too), it can be fantastic to lie back with them in skin contact and let them take their time to search out the breast.

Try to observe what skills your baby displays right from the very beginning, how their head bobs around with their mouth getting wider and wider, for example, and push with their feet, launching themselves up to find the breast. You can do this with them from moments after birth to any time in the first couple of months.

This laid-back feeding position, and baby-led latching, has been found to be much less likely to cause nipple pain and damage, so it's well worth trying it, to get off to a good start. And don't just feel you can only do it straight after birth – keep using it!*

However, you may equally find that it takes your baby quite some time to figure out how to latch and feed, and that they may not search for the breast straight away. This might be because of some impact from birth, such as medication or how they were born, for example, or sometimes it just simply takes some time. Please don't panic if they don't feed. As much as, yes, it would be great to have them feeding straightaway, it does *not* mean that you won't be able to breastfeed.

If they don't show feeding cues shortly after birth, you'll be encouraged to hand express some colostrum. Colostrum is the first milk your body produces (see p. 17 for more information). The reason you'll be encouraged to express if they don't feed is partly to give some colostrum to the baby, but it's also largely to stimulate your breasts and hormones. This helps kick start them into action in regards to getting your milk supply up and running.

This is one of those moments in life when timing matters: your hormones are doing some special stuff behind the scenes in those first few days, and you need to be on it with the expressing from the beginning to tell your body it needs to set up for a full milk supply. This can be a real challenge, especially if you haven't hand expressed before, so learning about hand expressing before your baby is born is a really good idea.

---

* For more about this, and how best to hold your baby to feed well, refer to the section on position and latching on p. 42.

Why hand expression and not pumping? Well, that's because it's much more effective for colostrum, the thick and sticky first milk, which would likely get stuck to the pump's sides. Colostrum is made in small amounts, so it's easier to collect by hand than pump. If they're able to, sometimes parents even hand express in the last weeks of their pregnancy, in order to freeze some colostrum in advance (don't worry, you can't use it up), in case they find themselves in a situation where the baby needs colostrum but they're unable to provide it, or want to have extra on hand. But hand expressing is also a fantastic, useful technique to learn, that will come in handy again and again throughout your breastfeeding journey (see p. 134 for more about it).

Colostrum – the first milk

- Concentrated amounts, just right for a new baby's tiny tummy.

- Laxative effect to help clear meconium (baby's first poo) and prevent jaundice (yellow colouring to the skin).

- Perfectly tailored to your baby.

- Starts being produced mid-pregnancy.

- Lines the immature gut so that germs are less likely to get into the bloodstream.

- Contains millions of germ-killing cells.

- Usually thick and sticky, but can be more watery too. Often yellow but can be clear.

The amount of colostrum you give to your baby in the first few hours will likely be very small, sometimes a matter of a few drops. And that's perfect.

If your baby is well and was born a healthy size, they will have special fat and energy stores that only newborns have, that ensure they're perfectly capable of managing with only small amounts of colostrum for a while. That said, it's important your baby is monitored if they're not feeding, to check they're doing okay, so speak with whomever is looking after you for support if you have any concerns.

> 'After Eli was born, she was put straight onto my chest. It was amazing how quickly she started searching for a feed. The midwives helped me get her latched on and she was feeding within 20 minutes!' – Olivia, mum of 2.

> 'Tobias had to go straight to the NICU after he was born and I couldn't hold him for the first 12 hours. I hand expressed every couple of hours until he was able to try and latch. He eventually fed at 16 hours old and it was such a relief!' – Lou, parent of 3.

The next feeds

After an initial period of activity, you may find your baby wants to crash out a bit, and you probably will too. Generally speaking, in that first 24 hours, a full-term baby of a healthy birth weight will need to feed or for you to express some colostrum every few hours or more. Some babies will wake for feeds, others will need to be woken. Some will be quite hesitant to feed, and while that may be normal, it's worth getting them checked over by a midwife (or whoever is caring for you). If your baby was born small, early, or has any risk factors for becoming unwell, you'll be encouraged to make sure they feed well and often, and a plan should be discussed with you about what will happen if they don't. Remember: hand-expressing colostrum is the most beneficial thing you can do here, and lots of skin contact where possible.

Feeding cues

How do you know when a baby wants to feed? Well, you might be surprised to hear that it's not about crying. Crying is actually the very last in a series of different cues they exhibit to show they want to feed.

So what are you looking for? With a newborn, basically any sort of body activity is a sign they want to feed! Check out the box below for a list.

Feeding cues

Rooting (searching with their mouth opening and closing)

Turning head side to side

Licking

Sucking fingers/putting hand into mouth

Body wriggling and stretching

Nappies

In the first 24 hours, we expect a baby to pass their first wee and poo. Ideally one to two or more wet nappies, and at least one poo.

This first poo is called meconium, and will be thick and very dark coloured, often appearing black – it's actually a very dark green. It doesn't usually have a smell to it, thankfully! But it can be quite messy.

Top tip: because it's tar-like and sticky, cotton wool balls are rarely effective at getting it off, and baby wipes can be harsh on a newborn's skin. Try using reusable wipes or flannels instead to get the bulk of it off, and cotton wool pads for the rest.

The second day

At this point, you may be putting the baby to the breast when they wake, you may be waking them to feed, they may never have gone to the breast, or they may be doing a mix of feeding and having expressed colostrum. All are very common.

Although it may feel like they've been here on the outside for a long time by now and that you should know what you're doing, in reality they're still very *very* new and you're both only in the very early days of learning how all this works. Try not to put too much pressure on yourself – although it can be very frustrating, there's still lots and lots of time to get things sorted. The most important things you can do are those skin-to-skin cuddles, feeding/offering frequently, and hand expressing if needed. Doing these things will 'keep the doors open' for establishing feeding. This is new for both of you.

You may find that sometimes your baby latches well; you may find others are sore – this is common, but not normal. You may well have heard that feeding shouldn't be painful if your baby is latched deeply, but, in reality, it takes all of us some time to get the latch perfected, so some soreness can happen. What's important to note, though, is that pain, soreness, cracks and bleeding very much shouldn't be brushed off as normal and to be expected. So while this sort of thing can happen, the aim is to try to keep adjusting the latch and position, or looking for the underlying cause, not just putting up with it. Please, please don't just put up with it because Auntie Barbara told you it's normal for your nipples to fall off!*

The second night

Oooof, this is a toughy – not gonna lie! 'Second night syndrome' is a common phenomenon where new babies on their second night after birth sort of wake up to the world and decide they want to feed and feed and feed. Unfortunately, it often coincides with when your excitement over the birth starts to calm down and you crash a bit and decide you really need some sleep, and it's sometimes your first night home from hospital too – leaving you worrying that it's all starting to unravel and go wrong.

But try not to worry, as 'second night syndrome' is actually a really positive sign. And when you know it's coming, it's easier to cope with, which is why I mention it here.

Babies usually settle a bit more in the morning, so try to catch up on some sleep then. And make sure you're not organising lots of visitors. I know it's a really exciting time and you're desperate to show your baby off, but I promise you that keeping things calm and quiet will be beneficial to you, and, just as importantly, beneficial to establishing breastfeeding too.

---

* See p. 43 for more information about latching and how to get this sorted.

Thinking back to when Covid first hit here in the UK, we had no idea how bad it was, and we didn't even know if we could touch the post pushed through the door by the postie. No one was allowed in your house, even health professional visits were suspended unless it was life or death. While this was really tough, of course, what I found was that a significant number of the families I was working with (over Zoom, of course!) actually enjoyed not having the pressure of family and friends traipsing through; that having that taken away from them, guilt free, meant they were able to focus on their basic needs, and that's *so* important. Staying in bed, eating, sleeping, feeding, resting and relaxing – bonding! These are *the* most important things right now. Everything else can, and will, wait, I promise.

And if you do have people come round, make sure they bring food, do something helpful, and only stay for a really short time.

> *'On the second night, Amera just wouldn't settle. She wanted to be on my boob constantly. It was reeeeally hard and I was so tired I reached several points where I didn't think I could go on. About 4am I hit breaking point and my other half took her and walked the floors for half an hour while I had a sleep. I wouldn't have thought it would help, but, actually, just that small sleep kept me going until morning, when she settled a lot better. I'm so glad I pushed through that night. But I wish I'd had more snacks in!'* – Claire, mum of 1.

Second-day nappies

Frequent feeding on that second night, as we've discussed, can be very normal, especially if you're finding it's comfortable. But keep an eye on those nappies to double check all is well. You're expecting at least two poos, and at least two wees. The poo is

22

likely to still be dark in colour, though you may start to notice a new lighter colour creeping in.

You may also see a dark, rust-coloured staining in the wee in the nappy; it can occasionally look like blood at first glance and be a bit scary! This staining is caused by small crystals called urates. For some babies it is normal – for others, though, it can be a sign that they need a little more milk. So go back to basics with position and latch to make sure they're feeding as effectively as they can and feeding frequently, and perhaps consider offering some expressed colostrum too. Discuss with your midwife for support with this.

Sometimes, with girls, there will be a small amount of blood in the nappy or around the vulva. This is a little like a baby period, and is to do with withdrawal from maternal hormones, which the baby was exposed to in the womb. It isn't a problem and usually only happens for a day or so. Of course, if you're worried, get it checked out.

Jaundice

If you spot any yellowing to their skin, or the whites of their eyes, contact your maternity triage for support. In the first 24 hours, this would be an emergency and you need to get your baby seen straight away.

In the following few days, however, some jaundice *may* be normal, especially if a baby has had some bruising during birth, but it can also be a sign they're not feeding as effectively as needed and need support to take more milk.

Jaundice is not something you would be particularly expected to notice, which is why the midwife visits are timed so that they can keep an eye out for stuff like this, but if you happen to think your baby is a bit yellow – like a bad fake tan – talk to your midwife.

If your baby becomes sleepier and reluctant to feed, seek support urgently.

Days three to five

Around days three to five after birth is when people talk about your milk 'coming in'. In reality, you've had milk for a long time: colostrum is milk! And the amounts of colostrum gradually increase as the hours and days go by. But there is a day, usually between Day 3 and Day 5, where you'll notice your breasts suddenly feel a lot fuller and heavier, and you might think 'ohhhkay, *now* I've got milk'. What's happened is that the amount of milk you're producing has increased, but also the composition of the milk has changed slightly, to match what your baby now needs. This means that you may start to notice some different, and sometimes more obvious signs during feeding.

You'll probably be able to recognise when they're swallowing more easily, for example, such as slightly slower sucks with deeper chin drops. Often this is a loud affair, but even if it isn't, there are signs you'll be able to recognise. Frequent swallowing means drinking well!

You'll also feel that each breast feels fuller and heavier before a feed, and that it will have softened after. Not fully softened, because you'll probably have some inflammation (swelling) of the breast tissue as well as the increased milk, but they should be noticeably softer, because a lot of the milk is now in the baby. And because that milk is now in the baby, they will often be more

24

settled after a feed. Parents often talk about the 'milk drunk' look. They come off the breast and look incredibly satisfied and snoozy, like they've had a few too many sherries with Christmas lunch and have fallen asleep in front of *Home Alone 3*.

In these first days, with the bigger milk volumes, breasts can sometimes feel very hard and full. Partly because of the larger volumes of milk, but partly because of swelling. See p. 115 for more information about engorgement and a technique called reverse pressure softening that can help.

If you've been hand expressing for feeds, now is a good time to start pumping, if you'd like to do so. If hand expressing is working well for you, that's fine too. The milk you're producing from this point onwards tends to resemble more recognisable 'milk', and pumping can be effective (see p. 138 for more about pumping).

You may also find that you can change how you give the expressed milk to a different method. You may have been using a feeding syringe (there's no needle, don't worry!) and might now consider using cup feeding, or occasionally a bottle.

Day Three to Five Nappies

More milk going into the baby also means more coming out the other end.

Their wees will change, not only in frequency, but also the amount of wee, the colour and maybe even the smell. Wee should start to become more clear or light straw-coloured, and not smell strongly (NB: if the wee smells strongly, like when you walk past a set of urinals, that's often a sign they're a bit dehydrated and need more milk).

A general guide is that you'll see at least one wee for each day of life for the first six or seven days. So Day Two: two wees, Day Four: four wees etc. But once your 'milk is in', you'll likely get more quite quickly, and the nappies will feel much heavier and fuller. It should feel as if you've gone from throwing a couple of teaspoons of water into the nappy, to several tablespoons.

Of course, the wee may not go into the nappy at all. Babies really do like to bless you with a wee the minute you remove the nappy! Top tip: keep a stack of towels handy next to where you're going to be changing nappies, especially for baby boys, who will delight in showing you their best impression of a fountain. And when putting a fresh nappy on a boy, always point their penis down!

Poo will start to change about now too: first to a lighter green or brown colour, then through to yellowy, and it may have seed-like bits in it. This is how the poo will then stay, for the most part, until your baby starts solid food. It has a sweet sort of yeasty smell. At least two in 24 hours is important as a sign of getting enough milk, but some babies will poo much more frequently, sometimes even after every feed!

> 'On Day 3, mid-morning, I went for a nap. When I woke up my boobs felt like they belonged to someone else. All of a sudden, they felt much bigger, much firmer, and they were quite tender, actually. I did find it quite reassuring, though, to feel them go softer after the babies had fed.' – Lisa, mum of twins Mildred and Herbie.

> 'The evening of Day 4, my chest was so hard I couldn't get baby to latch at all. It was like he had nothing to grip on to. I called the midwives, and they told me to look up something

26

called Reverse Pressure Softening and to hand express a bit to help too. I was then able to get him to latch' – Ash, parent of Seb.

Weight check

Your baby will usually be weighed on Day 3 or 5. Have a look at p. 94 for information about what to expect.

Conclusion

During these first few days, be kind to yourself. Eat well, and frequently. Drink plenty of water. Not because it'll impact how much milk you make directly, but because you're healing, you're tired, and you need stamina and energy.

Remember to take painkillers if you're in pain from your birth, as there are plenty that are compatible with breastfeeding. If pain is from feeding, though, get help promptly.

You may be in hospital, you may be home, depending on multiple factors. Sometimes you come home and go back again. But remember that, whatever happens, keeping up skin-to-skin snuggles wherever you can, and continuing to express milk, will keep the doors open to establishing breastfeeding.

I know it's all a bit of a whirlwind, but you'll do just great.

Sarah's story

I had my eldest daughter when I was twenty-three, and split up with my boyfriend during my pregnancy, ending up living back with my parents. I had lots of support, but as I sat in the hospital bed the night after she was born, watching this tiny, brand new person breathing in my arms, I felt very alone.

While I was pregnant I had thought I might try and breastfeed, but was surprised how much I wanted to make it work once she arrived. I had read some books about it, but at 3am in the hospital with only one thin pillow, it felt impossible. I wish I'd been assertive enough to ask for some support or at least a couple more pillows! We made it through that night, though, had a good few goes at feeding and it seemed to be working. Once we got home, we had a flurry of visitors and the days were good. I was getting very sore, but my grandma said it was just my nipples toughening up, so I wasn't too worried. It seemed like it was some kind of rite of passage and people nodded knowingly when they saw me wince and squirm as she latched on. After three or four days, it got to the point where I was having to brace myself before latching her on because there would be ten seconds of 'owwww!' At night, when we were alone, I began to dread it. I was feeling a strange mix of joy, pride, dread and guilt. Quite a spicy selection of emotions for a tired person! Eventually, after a particularly bad night around eight days in, where it seemed like my nipple was going to come off, we began to get into a routine. Together, we found positions that were comfy for us and I was reassured that she was gaining weight and getting gorgeously chubby. A few people started saying I should give her a bottle 'before she gets too used to breastfeeding', but she wasn't having any of it. After a few failed attempts, I accepted that we were going to be an exclusively breastfeeding twosome and made my peace with it. Looking back on it now, those quiet, night-time feeds were such precious moments for us and, in all honesty, I think I'm too lazy for bottle feeding – no equipment or prep required for boobing! So it's probably a good thing that she didn't fancy the idea of a bottle. Eventually, my daughter self-weaned at 14 months, and our family later grew, but I'll always remember that first year when it was just us two and we were everything to each other.

3

How to feed your baby!

'Lucy, what do you mean *how*? You just stick a boob in their mouth, right?'

'Fraid not.'

This bit right here really is one of the keys to happy breastfeeding, but it can also be one of the trickiest parts. Learning how to get your baby effectively feeding in a comfortable way takes time and patience, whether it's your first baby or your tenth.

'But it's natural!' Yes, but it's natural like walking, not like breathing. It's a learned skill. It isn't quite as easy as pop a nipple in their mouth and off you go; there is a specific way they need to be held and latched to the breast for things to go well.

Give yourself lots of time, be patient but determined, and remember to go easy on yourself while you're learning. You'll get there, but it does take practice.

Let's break it down . . .

What is positioning?

Positioning is the term you may hear that describes how you hold your baby to allow them to feed effectively. It's basically how you hold their body close to you to feed well, but there's lots of different ways people do it.

What is latching?

Latching (or sometimes attachment) is how the baby takes the breast into their mouth to then transfer (drink) the milk. Or, basically, how they've got their chops on the boob.

It's *so* important!

A baby that is positioned and latched well on the breast will be able to drink the milk they need, when they need it. This means your baby will be much happier, and that means you will be too. It also means they're less likely to be unsettled with things like trapped wind, and reflux, which we'll talk about later on in the book. So fewer hours pacing the floor wondering what's wrong, basically.

Plus, the more milk they take, the more you make. Milk supply mainly works on supply and demand. So an effective latch is also really important for making just the right amount of milk, both for now but also for the long run too as your baby grows.

When they're latched well, the feed will be comfortable for you, and your breasts and nipples will stay pain and damage free. Sounds good, huh?!

How do I do it? Positioning

There are lots of names used for different positions, such as cross cradle, or koala hold, but do you need to know the names to breastfeed? Nah, not really.

What you *could* do with knowing, though, is that there are key things to remember no matter whether your baby is across your front, lying next to you, or round your side.

I like to call these the four Ts – Turn, Tug, Tuck, Tilt. This is not an official thing at all, it's just me, Lucy, trying to find a way to help you remember it! Let me explain:

Turn – Turn your baby in toward you.

Tug – Tug them in the direction of their feet.

Tuck – Tuck their bottom in.

Tilt – Tilted-back head.

Let me expand on the four Ts a bit more:

Turn your baby toward your body –
Try this yourself as you sit or stand there: twist your neck round to the side, chin over your shoulder. Try swallowing a few sips of a drink. Not easy! Now turn your head back straight so that your hips, body and neck and chin are all in line, try that swallowing again. Much easier! This is why the baby needs to be turned in to match you. Not only is it more comfortable for them, but they'll be able to feed much more effectively.

Tummy to mummy? This phrase used to be used a lot and you may still hear it. It's catchy, which is handy, but doesn't work quite so well for those parents whose nipples point more downward. You'll need to adjust your baby's position for your own anatomy, depending on how big or small your boobs are, where your nipples are positioned and which way they angle. So please do have a play around with angles until you find the right one for you. Keep in mind that it's best if the baby is not twisted in any way, so check their chin, shoulders, body and hips are in a straight line, and hold them into you really close no matter which position you use.

Tug them in the direction of their feet –
Okay, okay, you don't actually have to tug them, but moving them round your body in the direction of their feet is actually really helpful. By doing this, it means your baby will start with the nipple up by their nose or even their eyes, which may seem ridiculous when you're trying to get the breast in their mouth! But babies open their mouths not by lowering their chin down, but by levering up their top jaw. So if the nipple is up by their nose, when the top jaw lifts up and their mouth is open, the nipple will then be pointing at the back of the roof of their mouth, which is the perfect spot to bring them forward for the latch.

Tuck their bottom in –
Your baby needs to be held really close against your body. If they're not close, they won't be able to get a deep mouthful. By tucking their bottom into you, not only will they be nice and close, but they're at a really good angle to get the right latch (where the nipple aims for the back of the roof of the mouth). Make sure their arms aren't between your bodies either – try to have an arm out either side of your baby's torso, in a sort of 'superman' arms pose, or a boob hug. If their arm is between you, then they're not able to get close enough in.

Effective, comfortable position

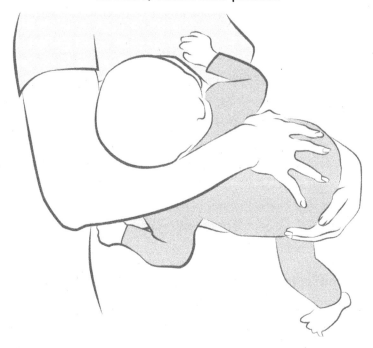

Ineffective, uncomfortable position

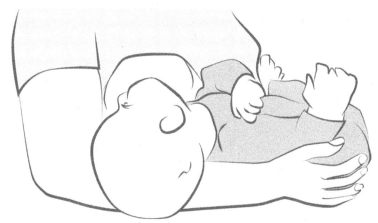

Tilt their head back (NB: you don't tilt their head back, they do) –
Your baby needs to be able to tilt their head back to latch well. This means making sure you don't have anything in the way of their head tipping back, no hand on the back of their head, not even a finger, no pillow in the way . . . I know, you've spent your whole life being told to protect the baby's head and then I come along and tell you to let it go! But, actually, as long as they've got good support for their shoulders and neck, they're absolutely fine. Don't forget that they've got reflexes encouraging them to do this.

Try this: point your finger straight forward at your mouth, open your mouth by keeping your chin where it is and tipping your head back and then push your finger forward and see where it hits. Tongue, right?

This time, point your finger angled towards your nose, tip your head back the same way again and push your finger in. See how far it goes back?

That's where the nipple needs to be. Right at the back of the mouth by the soft palate.

If your baby feels all wobbly and unstable, try leaning yourself back just a bit. If you're sitting, try shuffling your bottom forward in the chair; you might need to put a cushion behind your lower back to support you, then relax back into it. Taking a bit more of your baby's body weight into your body rather than through your wrist can really help you feel confident to leave their head free.

Uncomfortable, avoid hand on back of head

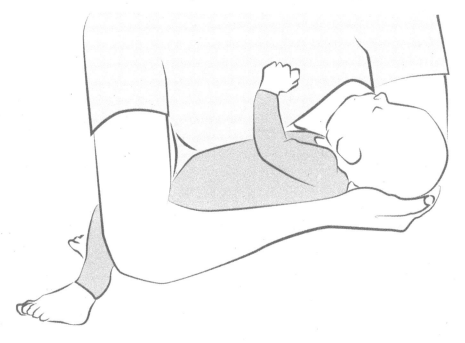

Comfortable, supporting shoulders and neck

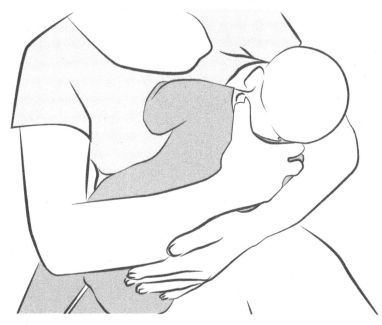

Cradle Hold

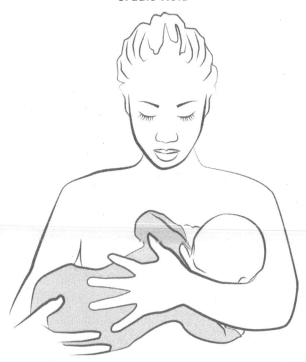

Cross Cradle

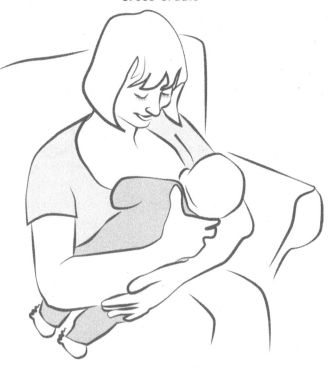

Laid Back from above

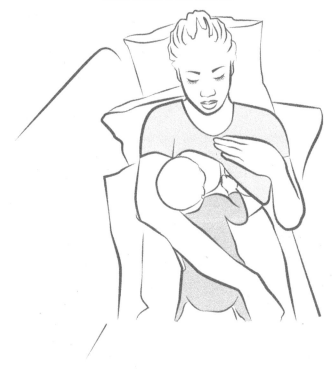

Laid Back side view

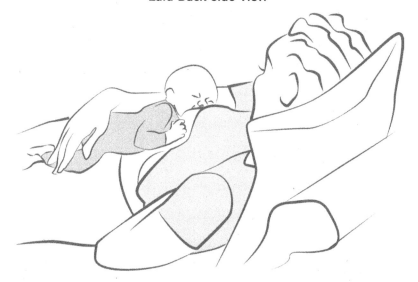

Rugby Hold

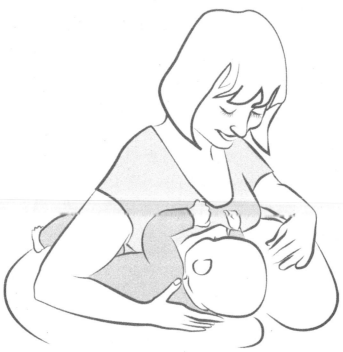

Side Lying

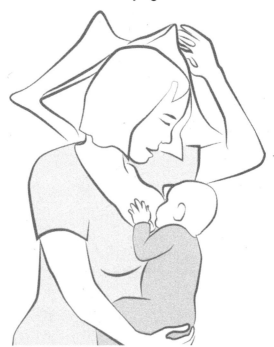

Pillows

Should I use a breastfeeding cushion?

You can, of course, but you don't need to. Ideally, you want to latch the baby first, and then use cushions or pillows afterwards for support if needed, otherwise they can get in the way of their head tipping back, or may position the baby at the wrong height for a comfy feed. You can use any cushions you have available, but some people prefer a specific feeding pillow.

Hands keep getting in the way?

Oh those hands!! You're all lined up for the perfect latch and then: bang! A hand pops in the way. Or you can't even get a position sorted because they're just kneading away with their little paws.

See, babies have very limited vision and use all their senses to find their way to latch well. Those little hands that can prove so tricky during latching are actually helping your little one figure out where they are and what's going on. It may seem like it's random movements, but it's telling them a lot. Keeping their hands bare helps them find their way, so ditch the scratch mitts and the swaddle when you're feeding.

If their hands are making things incredibly difficult, however – which can definitely happen – there are a couple of things to consider.

First, getting their chin onto your breast. If you feel like they're flailing around a bit and seeming quite lost, it can be helpful to get their chin forward onto your breast. That connection of chin to skin will often be enough to make them relax those arms and hands enough to get latched, a little like they've found their target!

41

Secondly, trying a different position. If you're using a position where they're lying on their side, it can be common for hands to get in the way. It seems that in these positions babies are more likely to feel a bit unstable and so their arms and hands can seem to desperately seek to stabilise themselves. If you want to stay in this position, do what you can to help them feel stable. Is their bottom tucked in tightly to you and supported? Do they need something against their feet? Does leaning back just a little help gravity secure them close against your body so they relax?

Alternatively, try a position where you're more laid back, which can allow a more baby-led attachment, or, alternatively, a 'koala hold', which is more upright and can help with a stable feeding. See p. 38–40 for other holds.

> 'I found the traditional positions of holding her across my body just so fiddly. I couldn't seem to support her right and her hands were in the way and we usually just ended up sweating and crying and putting up with a rubbish latch, terrified to remove her and try again.
>
> Then someone showed me the koala hold and it was a game changer. I felt much more comfortable supporting her that way; my arms weren't aching, she seemed happier and wasn't wind-milling her arms around getting them in the way as much.'
>
> 'It was so painful doing it the way I was shown in hospital, but I put up with it thinking it was what I had to do. Then a midwife assistant came to my house and got me lying down and sort of plopped Ben on top of me. Gravity seemed to help loads and he was able to wriggle until he was in a comfier spot. It was nice for me to be able to rest as well. I was worried that I wouldn't be able to feed like that outside of my home,

but as time went on we were able to get more confident using other positions for out and about' – Gabby, mum to Ben.

How do I do it? Latching

Once your baby is in a position that is going to allow them to latch well, you'll see that they'll probably be able to open up really wide to reach for a big mouthful of breast. And this is important, it is *breast* feeding, not nipple feeding. We're not just trying to get the nipple in their mouth here.

So, first of all, you've got them in a nice straight line, turned in and really close to you, nothing in the way of the back of their head, and your nipple is high up their face. You might be supporting your breast with your hand, or you may not need to. If you do, make sure you're not moving your breast at all, but letting it sit where it naturally sits, and keep your fingers well out of the way of your nipple and areola.

When they tip their head back and open really wide, their tongue will be down and ready to scoop up the breast, and the nipple will be pointed at the back of the roof of the mouth. That's when you swiftly bring them forward by the shoulders and they will latch.

Bring them to you, not you to them. Let them do the work, don't try and 'post' your nipple into their mouth.

Where does the baby's bottom lip need to be and why?

To get a deep, comfortable, effective latch, the baby needs to come to the breast at an angle that you might not expect. They don't come onto the breast centrally, like the nipple is a target, but at an angle that looks more 'wonky'.

In order to get this 'asymmetric latch', it's important to look at the baby's bottom lip. The reason we talk about 'nose to nipple', or having the nipple lined far up the baby's face, is actually so that their bottom lip starts, and stays, well away from the base of your nipple.

If you imagine the bottom lip is Velcroed or superglued to that spot, the rest of the latch will fall beautifully into place.

You'll be able to see more of your areola above the baby's nose than by their chin. More moustache than beard!

Coming onto the breast

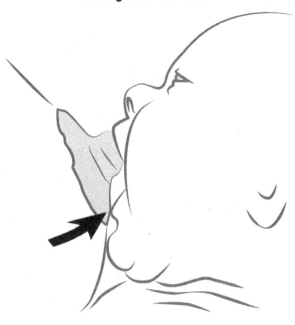

Unlatching

If you need to unlatch them to try again, use your little finger and either pull back on their cheek slightly, or gently manipulate it into the corner of their mouth. This will break the suction and you can then pull them off.

Keep clean hands, sucking your finger first won't make it any cleaner!

At first, trying to coordinate latching will feel like trying to learn to play the drums drunk and blindfolded. But you'll get it sorted! Give yourself time. It is absolutely not just you that finds this tricky, it *is* tricky!

How can I tell they're latched well?

So you've managed to get them latched: well done! Take a deep breath and relax your shoulders. Now let's have a look and see how things are, but don't prod and poke to see as this can shift the latch. Just look. There are some signs you can watch out for that will help you figure out if things are going well.

First, it should feel *comfortable*. Okay, the first ten seconds or so may feel a bit ouchy, especially in those early days, but after ten seconds or so it should calm down and be pain free. If it's not, something isn't quite right and you may need to relatch. Frustrating for sure! But worth doing, I promise.

Your nipple should come out the same shape it went in, just perhaps a bit longer. If it looks pinched, flattened or misshapen in any way, that shows it's been getting compressed in the baby's mouth and the latch needs adjusting.

Signs of a deep latch

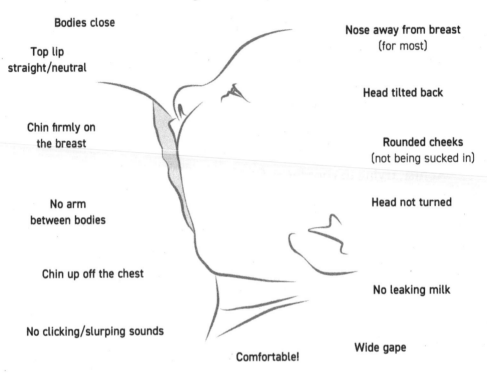

Bodies close

Top lip straight/neutral

Nose away from breast (for most)

Head tilted back

Chin firmly on the breast

Rounded cheeks (not being sucked in)

No arm between bodies

Head not turned

Chin up off the chest

No leaking milk

No clicking/slurping sounds

Comfortable!

Wide gape

Lip blisters

Sometimes new babies get blisters on their lips. This is common, but not normal as such. It shows they're using their lips to grip on, which shouldn't need to happen if the latch is deep enough. A blister in the middle of their top lip is usually a sign of needing some position and latch changes. Blisters all along the top lip, known as 'cobblestones' because of their appearance, often signal difficulties with oral restriction, such as tongue tie.

If everything else is going well, and blisters are the only thing you've noticed that seem a bit off, check the four Ts, and/or visit a peer support group in your local area and talk it through, but please don't worry, as the blisters won't harm your baby.

Fast milk flow

For some parents, especially in the early days, you can feel like you've got quite a fast flow, or that the first release of milk (the 'let down') is pretty forceful. The baby may come off the breast and cough and splutter, and you might find your milk spraying across the room!

You can help a baby cope with this fast flow by making sure they have a deep, asymmetric latch. Most babies can cope with even the fastest of flows as long as it's hitting the right spot in their mouth and not directly at the back of their throat.

The first port of call is always to go back to basics with position and latch; try some self-attachment in a skin-to-skin cuddle. If your baby can't latch any deeper, or if they're still struggling despite changes, there are a few other things you can do: you can catch the milk in a muslin, towel, or container and wait until the sprays have subsided before latching them on; or you can try an upright position, such as koala hold, or a laid-back position to keep gravity in your favour and slow that milk flow! Fast flow can be more spectacular when your breasts are fuller, so feeding frequently, especially in the early days, helps to manage this. You may also find that fast flow is a bigger issue at some times of the day and not an issue at all at others, and this is very normal. For most, fast flow issues in the early days calm down a lot as your milk supply regulates and settles to your baby's needs. Most parents only need to follow their baby's feeding cues and feed often for this to happen.

Flipple technique

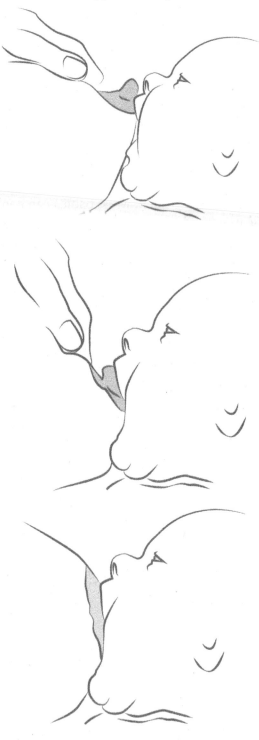

The 'flipple' and breast shaping

What triggers a baby's sucking reflex is the nipple hitting right at the back of the roof of their mouth. So, if your nipple is flatter or inverted, it can be trickier to get that to happen. In this situation, it can be helpful to use some breast shaping or a nipple flick or 'flipple' technique.

To shape your breast to allow deeper latching, you cup your breast and squeeze your fingers and thumb together on opposite sides just about two or three inches back from your nipple. It's a little like squashing a really big sandwich down a bit to allow you to get more in your mouth.

The nipple flick, or 'flipple' technique, is where you use a thumb or finger on the side of your breast and push in or pull back slightly, to angle your nipple further away from the baby. This creates a bump of breast on the opposite side where your baby's lower lip will be. When they open wide, you then push the thumb or finger you're using forward to flick the nipple much further into their mouth. You then lift the baby to you, taking care to make sure that you really do lift the baby to you, and that the nipple flick doesn't turn into you leaning forward and posting the nipple into baby's mouth. Remember: we need to keep that bottom lip far away from the base of the nipple.

What about shields?

For babies that are struggling to latch because they can't get deeply enough onto the breast, nipple shields are sometimes suggested. Nipple shields are a thin silicone cover for the nipple, a little like a sombrero. Because they protrude far, they can be really helpful with allowing the baby to get hold and start feeding.

However, they come with pros and cons, so it's definitely something that should be discussed fully before you consider using them. Read more about nipple shields on p. 79.

Conclusion

I know you might be reading this and thinking you'll *never* get the hang of breastfeeding, but you will. It's so common for parents to say to me that they don't know how they'll ever be out there meeting a friend for coffee and managing to feed effortlessly. But you have to give yourself time, be patient, and keep determined and confident that you *will* get it. It's entirely normal for it to take some time, even weeks or longer, for this bit to get sorted. Hugely frustrating, I know, but in reality that's what it's like for many parents. It's a bit like learning to drive: at first there's so much stuff to coordinate and it's a conscious effort that takes time, but after a while you just get in the car and go . . .

If something doesn't feel right, or it's not working, keep asking for help and trying different things. Sometimes just the smallest movement or adjustment, even a matter of millimetres, can make all the difference.

Get yourself along to a local support group if you can too, as often the other parents there and the peer supporters can really help. And, before you know it, *you* will be that parent sitting feeding like a natural in the café with someone pregnant glancing at you wondering how on earth you're doing it!

Emma's story

My little boy, Patrick, was born at 7am. We had the whole day together in the maternity unit and I was determined to go home that evening.

Patrick struggled to latch from the off; the midwives and breast-feeding support team came and he just wasn't getting it. We tried all sorts of different positions with no joy, so we decided to wait a little while and try later. While on our own I got what I thought was a good feed – in hindsight it wasn't – and so we were discharged based on my telling them we were all good.

Breastfeeding was so, so difficult for us. I have large boobs and my nipples did not want to protrude, meaning that Patrick just couldn't get a latch. I bought nipple shields, tried making my nipples cold or pumping before a feed, but nothing really worked. We got advice from a friend who is a lactation consultant and also our NCT lactation guide, who were both great, but no joy. In all the videos I had seen of breastfeeding, the mums' nipples were sticking out and mine never did that, so I thought I was doing something wrong.

After about a week I was a mess; every feed was ending in tears for both of us. So I stopped. I kept pumping, as I wanted him to have my milk, but I stepped away from breastfeeding directly. It was exhausting, as every feed became double the length – pumping after I had fed the baby.

About ten days after stopping, I was in the bath with Patrick and my husband suggested we give it another try. We were both really relaxed, having lots of skin on skin, and there was no pressure about making it work. After a few false starts, Patrick latched like he had been doing it for ever and fed. So we tried it a few more times in the bath and slowly worked our way back up to every feed over the next few weeks.

It would have been so easy to not have restarted, but we are now five months down the line and I love the connection my little man and I have during our feeding sessions. He still takes a bottle from Dad, but most feeds are from the breast.

I hope that my story shows that breastfeeding has to work for *both* of you and that it is okay to stop. But also that taking a step away doesn't mean you can't come back to it.

4

How do I know they're getting enough milk?

For a lot of us, this is a real worry. What if, no matter how much we want to breastfeed, and how hard we try, we just don't have enough milk?

The thing is, society has drummed it into us that we're somehow not enough for our babies, that we need loads of products and stuff. Almost every baby doll we can buy for children comes with a bottle, for example, so arguably we grow up with the subliminal message that we won't be able to make enough milk, and that this is the norm. It seems like everyone you meet when you're pregnant has a story about not having enough milk, doesn't it? Along with the adverts for bottles and formula everywhere, it can make you feel like insufficient milk is an inevitability. But it's not!

For the vast majority of people, there is no problem with the amount of milk they make at all, but, nevertheless, the possibility niggles at the back of our minds. So when something comes along, like our breasts feel softer suddenly, or our baby wants to feed a lot more, we get totally thrown, and convinced our milk supply is plummeting.

Let me tell you a secret: it usually isn't. Honestly.

There's a lot of things that happen with breastfeeding and new babies that can make us feel like things are going wrong, but when you can understand what's happening and how to cope, it can help reassure you that, actually, it's normal. And if it's *not* normal, understanding what's going on helps you know how and where to seek support.

This chapter will have a look at how to recognise they're getting enough milk, as well as some of the common reasons parents may feel they're not – and what's *actually* going on.

Comfortable feeds

If feeding is comfortable for you, that's a really reassuring sign! Remember: you're working as a team, you and your baby. So if you're not comfortable, then something isn't right. And I'm not just talking about nipple comfort either, but comfortable for your whole body. Go back to the 'How to feed your baby' chapter to troubleshoot, and the nipple and breast pain chapter, if adjusting latch isn't helping.

Position and latch

In chapter 3, we talked about the way the baby is positioned and latched has a massive impact on how much milk they can drink, so this is always one of the first things to think about if you're wondering if they're getting enough. If the latch is effective and comfortable, they're much more likely to be drinking well.

Always remember that going 'back to basics' along the way during your breastfeeding journey will help make sure things go well.

What goes in, must come out

'I never knew I would become so obsessed with my baby's poo. I even had a gallery on my phone of pictures!' – Sinita, mum of Obi.

Your baby's nappies will tell you a *lot* about what's going on. You'll see at least six heavy wet nappies and at least two poos in every 24 hours, from around five days old until six weeks, and this is a really reassuring sign that they're getting enough milk. From six weeks onward, you *may* see slightly less poo, and it may be normal for them, but it's still worth double checking all is well if they start to poo less frequently.* For the most part, their poo will be soft and yellow. Sometimes with seedy bits in it, sometimes without. Both can be normal.

Occasionally, you might get a different poo, such as a green one, or a watery one. And that's okay if it's the odd one. If a lot or all of the poos are different, though, it's a sign to get things checked out. An IBCLC would be a perfect person to speak to about this.

Frequency of feeds

Babies feed a *lot*. It's completely normal. They feed for hunger, for thirst, for comfort, for sleep, for connection, to pass wind . . . the list goes on and on! If your baby is feeding frequently, the chances are they *do* know what they're doing, but unfortunately we're not really set up to trust in that, and also there's a lot of pressure on us to get our babies independent pretty quickly (spoiler alert, you don't need to!).

---

* See the myths chapter for more info on poo frequency.

But frequent feeding really is something that you've just gotta go with most of the time and trust that it's okay. In those early weeks (and beyond), babies will usually feed at least eight to twelve times each 24 hours, if not more. And it's not a problem for them, or for feeding. But, wowsa! It's pretty tough for us. So make sure you've got lots of support around you, so you can spend a lot of time binge-watching TV and eating snacks (chocolate cravings are *real* during breastfeeding!).

Now, all this said, very frequent feeding *can* sometimes be a sign that something isn't quite right. So it's worth thinking about the rest of what's going on.

If there are any problems with their weight, or with the amount of wet and/or dirty nappies, or you have any other worries at all, connect with someone for a feeding assessment. It may be that there is something going on with milk supply, or it may be that it's to do with how the baby accesses the milk (their latch, for example). A well-trained supporter will be able to help you piece together what's happening and how to move forward.

What is a feeding assessment? (NB: it's not just a quick look at the latch!)

At every contact with a health professional you should be offered a feeding assessment.

This will include

- Watching a full feed together, from how baby latches on right to what happens at the end.

- Noticing how the latch looks and feels, including nipple shape after the feed.

- Sucking pattern.

- Noticing the suck/swallow frequency and helping you to recognise when they are actively drinking.

- Asking about nappy contents and frequency.

- Discussing how you're feeling about feeding and any worries you might have.

- Asking about frequency of feeds.

- Behaviour during and after feeds.

- Whether you use a dummy or any expressed milk or formula, why, and if you're happy with this.

- Discussing your concerns.

- Weight review (not every time).

Can I use a dummy?

Babies *love* to suck; it's soothing and comforting and one of their favourite things. Dummies or pacifiers have been used to soothe babies for a long time, and a lot of families still choose to use them now. There are, however, a few things to consider if you're opting to use one.

While some parents find breastfeeding is unaffected by the use of a dummy, for others it can have an impact on milk supply, weight gain, and/or latch. Because of this, it's important to try to wait until breastfeeding is well established before offering one, if that's what you wish to do.

If you're in the early days of feeding and feeling overwhelmed by the amount the baby wants to feed and considering using a dummy to help, it would be well worth getting a feeding review, if you can. They should be able to help you make sure feeding is as effective as it can be, and be able to assist you in avoiding a dummy, if you'd prefer.

Sucking and swallowing

There is a certain sucking pattern that babies go through when they feed, and this can be really helpful to watch for and recognise in your own baby.

When they first go onto the breast, they take quite quick sucks. These are stimulating and signal to your body: 'Hey, it's time for the milk please. boss'. Your body responds with a big wave of the hormone oxytocin (also known as the love hormone!). This causes your breast to release a surge of milk (the 'milk ejection reflex' or 'let down'), and you'll see that baby's sucking will change.

Now there will be deeper, more drawing sucks, with deeeeep chin drops just before they swallow (take a big mouthful of drink yourself and see how low your chin goes and then what happens when you swallow). You may even hear the swallow: it sounds like a little 'Kuh' sound!

It's also normal for a baby to take pauses through the feed and rest for a short while before starting again. You don't need to poke or stimulate them to get them going again (breast compressions can be helpful for babies that aren't transferring milk well, though – see p. 97 for more).

If they're feeding effectively, you'll be able to see that they take about one to two sucks before each swallow for the bulk of the feed. If they're doing lots of sucks between swallows often, or if they're having more pauses than bursts of sucking, it may be a sign that they're not transferring the milk effectively, or that your supply needs a bit of a boost.

What is 'let down'?

'Let down' is the name that people tend to use for when your milk starts to flow. It's actually a reflex, the 'milk ejection reflex' (MER) and it happens when your body decides to release the milk. Most often this is when the baby sucks (or you pump or hand express), but sometimes this can happen what feels like randomly – especially at first! You hear a baby cry, your arm brushes past your boob, you think about their little thumbs . . . whoosh, here comes the milk! It does become more of a conditioned response as time goes on, though, and your body ends up being quite sensible about when it lets the milk come.

If you're feeling tense, stressed or in pain, however, this can inhibit the milk from flowing. It makes sense, really; if you're in 'fight or flight' mode, your body knows it's probably not a good time to sit and feed. So if you take some deep breaths and relax your shoulders, perhaps do some breast massage, this can help get those hormones going and milk flowing.

Some parents feel a sensation with their 'let down', like tingling, pressure, pinching or something else. Sometimes it can be a bit uncomfortable, but this should only be for a few seconds.

Occasionally, the MER can cause a temporary wave of nausea, or some people experience a wave of negative emotion like sadness or despair. This is called DMER ('dysphoric milk ejection reflex') and can be very unpleasant. If you are experiencing this, you may benefit from talking therapies as well as feeding support.

Flutter sucking

Toward the end of the feed, you may notice your baby starts to suck more gently, and that the swallowing frequency slows down. This is often known as flutter sucking, because it feels a bit like fluttering! This is a very valid part of the feed, where they get comfort, and rest, start to digest their milk, and may even stimulate another milk ejection.

If you feel your baby moves to flutter sucking very quickly into a feed, though, for a lot of their feeds, speak with someone about a feeding assessment to check all is well.

Behaviour during feeds

At the beginning of a feed, a baby will often be a little bit wriggly and fractious as they try and stimulate the milk to flow. They may even come on and off a few times, and sometimes they even yell at the boob a bit! It can be really confusing when they're giving you signals that they want to feed and then start screaming at your boobs like they hate them. But, again, it's normal: don't worry!

Usually their fists will be balled, and up by their face (oh, those pesky hands getting in the way of latching!). They often bash at the boob too. You know how kittens knead while they feed? This is a bit like the human baby equivalent of that.

When the milk starts to flow, though, they tend to relax into the feed, and become more still. There's a very obvious kinda 'ahh, this is nice' to their body language.

This fidgetiness may come back toward the end of the feed as they try to stimulate more milk flow, or if they've got a bit of wind to process. Don't worry if this happens, but if they're unsettled at the breast a lot, it may be a sign that something isn't quite right.

Stimulating behaviours

There are certain behaviours that all babies do at some point to stimulate milk flow and supply and these can be normal. They happen more often during cluster feeding and growth spurts (see below).

Tugging. Chomping. Gumming down. Repeatedly latching on and off. Wriggling. Shaking their head from side to side. Pressing their face into the breast. Stroking. Hitting with their hands. Seeming like they can't find the nipple despite it being in their mouth.

What can help: revisit the four Ts, try some skin-to-skin cuddles, a bath together, and consider getting some skilled breastfeeding support.

Cluster feeding and growth spurts

'Cluster feeding' is the term given to when babies want to feed very frequently for several hours at a time. This is very common in the early weeks and months, and usually isn't a sign of a problem. It often happens in the evening, though not always.

It can happen even more during growth spurts, which are spells of a day or several days where a baby's need for feeds intensifies massively. It can be incredibly unnerving, but as long as their nappy output is good and feeding is comfortable, it's not usually a problem.

You will need support during this time, though, as it can be hard to do anything other than feed, eat and rest! Get a helpful friend or family member to do some laundry and bring you a massive pie.

Common times for growth spurts are around 10 days, 3–4 weeks, 6 weeks and 4 months. But they can happen at any time.

If you feel like your baby is cluster feeding too much, and growth spurts don't calm down after a few days, or you're worried about their nappy output at any point, reach out for help. In the meantime, go back to basics with position and latch, and get skin to skin.

Soft breasts

Soft breasts can make you worry that you don't have enough milk, or that your milk is drying up. In reality, soft breasts are a *good* thing! It shows that milk production is working well, and that your breasts are healthy and happy.

Full-feeling breasts actually signal to your body to slow milk production, so while it may feel reassuring that you've got a lot of milk in there right then, it's actually not great for supply.

Often, around the 10-day mark is when breasts first start to really soften down (don't worry if yours don't just yet, though), and combined with that first growth spurt, it can really unsettle you. But hang in there, and keep an eye on those nappies.

Let-down sensation

When the milk gets released by your body (i.e. 'milk ejection' or 'let down'), it can cause a sensation for some people. It may feel tingly, pinchy, like pressure, or warmth.

For some people, though, they don't feel anything and the only way they know it's happened is their little one is swallowing more! It's not a problem at all if you don't feel any sensation, as it's one of those strange differences between people, and doesn't signal a problem with supply.

It's also not an issue if you do have a sensation but then it disappears as the weeks or months go on; it's just another sign that your body is really comfortable with what it's doing.

Difficult evenings

Evenings with a new baby can be pretty tough, and often this kicks in around Week 2 or 3. They can seem unsettled and unhappy of an evening, and want to feed much more than usual (see cluster feeding, above).

Often your breasts can feel reeeeally soft at this time too, which can definitely make you feel like your baby is struggling to get enough milk. But this is actually incredibly common and rarely a problem (still difficult, though).

It seems like a combination of things often crop up around this time: firstly, not only are babies often tired and overstimulated, but we know that there are hormonal fluctuations for the parent over the 24 hours, and that evenings seem to be a bit of a low point. What this leads to is not only seemingly slower milk production, but also that sense that things feel more difficult. Anxiety and feeling overwhelmed are often reported by parents in the evening, and a common phenomenon known as 'bed dread' often takes place around now too.

> 'Evenings were really difficult for us in the first few months. Andrew would be so unsettled, wanting to be on the boob but then not being happy when he was there. Feeds felt more difficult and were relentless for hours. But then, around 11pm, he'd crash out for a few hours and everything would sort of reset. I used to feel so anxious and upset in the evenings, but by the middle of the night I felt fine again' – Sarah, mum of 1.

Leaking

Some parents find their breasts leak, others don't. Some have a mixture of both, or they start off leaking but then slow down and stop as the weeks or months go by.

Whether you leak or not is not an indication of your milk supply, though, so please don't worry if you're not soaking through breast pads.

If you are using breast pads, consider using washables. They're kinder to your skin, cheaper in the long run, and so much better for the environment.

Occasionally leaking can be excessive or annoying – if you find this, your local peer support group might be a good place to find practical solutions, and can help you find more help if you need it.

They won't be put down

Babies are not big fans of being put down, and tend to wake up from even the most settled of sleeps if you do try and pop them into your lovingly bought Moses basket!

When they wake, they usually start rooting and fussing immediately, and this request for a feed potentially so soon after another can make us worry they're not feeding well or not getting enough milk.

In reality, it's rarely to do with how much milk they're getting. Sure, sometimes they're genuinely hungry again, but, for the most part, it's a sort of protective mechanism and regulation tool. Let me explain: human babies are completely reliant on their caregiver. We're not like horses or sheep, able to get up and start walking around within minutes. We need absolutely all of our needs to be met by someone else. Food, warmth and comfort, sure, but also being kept safe from threats. So when they get put down human babies' immediate response is 'I'm alone, I'm not safe, I need latch back on and get myself sorted'.

So, no, it's not to do with not getting enough milk, but I totally get why it may feel like it.

This is really tough, though, because a baby wanting to be held nigh on 24/7 can often mean very little rest for you. So how do you survive it? Well, you need to rope in as much help as you can. If you've got a partner, share the load. Take it in shifts and have them hold the baby while you rest and vice versa.

This stage usually lasts up to two or three months, though it's not uncommon for it to go on longer. And this is one of those times when you really have to block out societal noise. The whole 'you have to put them down otherwise they'll only ever sleep on you' or 'you'll make a rod for your back' etc. People seem determined to scare us in these early months, to convince us that if we trust our babies to know what they need that we're somehow doing a negative thing. In reality, when we do what they need, it's so much easier. It's also really positive, because babies that are responded to and have their needs met have been found to be better attached to their parents, and to grow and develop more quickly and easily. This is not opinion, this is the evidence; no one has ever cuddled their baby too much and neither will you! They also tend to have better emotional health and development too. It really is the right thing to do, I promise.

Can't express much

If feeding is going well, then ideally you won't do any expressing in the first few weeks and will let your body regulate to what your baby needs. However, if you do choose to express for whatever reason, it's important to know that being able to express a large bottle of milk is most definitely not the norm. For most people, an ounce or two (30–60ml) is the most they'll get, if that. Please don't worry if you can't express much, as it really isn't an indication of your supply. The way a baby feeds and the way a pump works are very different, and on the whole babies are much more effective at removing milk.

> 'I've never been able to express; I just don't get on with it.
> The tiniest dribble in the bottom of the bottle, no matter what
> I do. But I've fed three babies and all have absolutely thrived!'
> – Laura, mum of 3.

Drinking a bottle after a breastfeed

Sometimes parents are so concerned their baby isn't getting enough milk that they choose to test this by offering a bottle. The baby then drinks the bottle and their worst fears are confirmed. But, actually, the reason the baby has drunk from the bottle may be nothing to do with hunger.

Sucking is a reflex. When something hits the roof of the mouth, the baby *will* suck; they can't stop themselves. Milk comes out of a bottle teat very easily, so when the baby sucks, milk flows into their mouth and they swallow. And repeat, and repeat, until eventually they fall asleep.

So, in actual fact, drinking from a bottle is a lot more about reflexes than hunger, and isn't an accurate test at all. If you get to the point of wanting to give a bottle because you're worried about hunger, it's well worth seeking some support to help you figure out what's really going on.

Weight gain

Of course, a good indicator that your baby is getting enough milk is if they're growing!* And don't forget that you don't need the scales to tell you if they are growing, as you'll be able to see it! They will physically get bigger as the weeks go by, and, before long, rapidly grow out of clothes (and nappies).

Conclusion

So many things can cause us to worry about whether our baby is getting enough milk, or about our milk supply. The idea that our bodies fail is deeply ingrained in our beliefs as a society, so don't be surprised if you have lots of nagging feelings about this.

But remember: a growing baby with full nappies is really reassuring!

If it turns out that there is a difficulty, it can usually be sorted, if that's what you would like. It doesn't have to be the end. There are many ways of improving breastfeeding and maxi-mising milk supply, and for those that don't make a full supply, combination feeding is an entirely valid option for many. Every drop of breastmilk is beneficial, and you're amazing. Don't *ever* forget that.

---

* Check out p. 93 for more information about weight gain.

Leez's story

Emily was my first baby. She was born ever so slightly early at 36+ weeks, but was a good weight at over 7lb. She passed her blood-sugar tests with no problems and we were able to go home from hospital after an overnight stay.

She always latched pretty well from the word go, I thought, and never had any problems with the amount of milk she was getting. She filled her nappies and grew very quickly.

At about ten days old, however, the midwife spotted that she had a very white tongue and questioned thrush. We got some drops for her, but it didn't make any difference. We eventually stopped giving them and it went away I think as her latch got better.

My husband had four weeks off work. When she was three weeks old, he had to go to his aunt's funeral overnight and I was home alone with the baby. It coincided with her first growth spurt too and it was a really rough night! But I made it through, albeit quite shaken.

I ate a *lot* of chocolate.

Evenings were very difficult with Emily. I'd feel extremely low and anxious, and she'd be very unsettled too. She'd want to feed a lot, but then fuss at the boob. We used to take it in 15-minute stints to hold and comfort her in the evenings so that neither one of us got too overwhelmed.

At about eight weeks she started to sleep longer stretches at night, about four or five hours, which felt wonderful. I started to add in some expressing in the morning because I felt quite full when we got up, but she would only want one side. I was going back to work at six months, so it felt useful to be able to store some for work.

Around ten weeks she started vomiting a lot more, which worried me. The GP suggested some sickness medication, but it didn't feel right to me, because she wasn't bothered by being sick and was generally happy and growing. She'd started chewing her hands and I realised I was offering the breast when perhaps she didn't need it, and she was overstuffing herself with milk. As I relearned her feeding cues, the vomiting calmed down a bit. She'd still puke after big feeds, but wasn't bothered, so I just had to learn to catch!

I'd say my biggest problem was my anxiety. So much of what happened for us was normal and okay, but I worried a lot. Looking back, I wish I'd been able to relax into it more. I wish I'd known where to get reliable help.

I loved breastfeeding her so much. It felt like this special, magical thing just between us two. I'm so glad I did it.

5

Nipple pain and problems

I sat having coffee with some of the school mums once, and we were talking about what we do for jobs. I tried to explain what I do and one said: 'Oh yeah, cracked bleeding nipples – I remember all that stuff', and they all nodded in agreement like it was just part and parcel of breastfeeding.

We've got ourselves in a bit of a pickle with this. Pain is common, but it's *not* normal. It's really not a terrible inevitability that you've got to get through, no matter what your Auntie Denise or the nipple cream companies might tell you. You do not have to put up with pain, and cracks, and bleeding!

And if anyone supporting you tells you 'your nipples just need to toughen up' or that you'll 'get used to it', then it's worth talking to someone else.

It's not anyone's fault that this has happened. You see, we've been a predominately bottle feeding society for generations, and we totally lost our way with breastfeeding. And now there's a load of mixed messages and bizarre advice that just won't seem to go away.*

---

* Have a look at the myths chapter for a breakdown of some of this stuff!

But in this chapter we'll talk about what might cause ongoing pain, and how to manage it.

Cracked nipples

The nipple is made to breastfeed, and it's perfect (yes, no matter what size or shape yours are). Just like feet are for walking on. But if they aren't looked after properly, they'll get damaged and painful. Just like if you crammed your feet into a small pair of shoes and walked for hours. So, just as finding the right size and shape pair of shoes is important for feet, so is finding the right position and latch for nipples!

As we touched on in the positioning section (see p. 32), if a baby isn't latched deeply onto the breast, or at the right angle, the nipple will get pinched and rubbed against the hard palate in the baby's mouth. Run your tongue back along the roof of your mouth now (or a finger, if you like) – you'll feel that it's hard and ridgey and then changes to soft and squishier. *This* is the place the nipple needs to be, the soft squashy bit. If it gets back there, it won't get compressed or rubbed, and it will be comfortable and remain undamaged.

The most common cause of cracked, damaged or painful nipples is how the baby is positioned and latched to feed. Adjusting this so that the baby comes on with a really wide gape, and the nipple gets right back to that soft spot, will make an instant difference for most. I know it can be really tricky working on that deep latch where everything feels okay, but you absolutely can do it.

It can make you feel really quite down and demoralised some-times, when you're having nipple pain, and you know it's coming from the latch but you just can't seem to change it. But keep

72

going, keep asking for support, and remember that lots of skin-to-skin laid back cuddles is often the way forward.

If you've been told the 'latch looks good' but you're still experiencing pain, cracks, or misshapen nipples, ask someone else, and someone else, and someone else again to help. The reason I say this is that, unfortunately, lots of parents get told their latch is perfect when actually there is a lot that needs adjusting. It shouldn't be this way, and I'm sorry that it is – I wish I could change it I really do!

Occasionally, cracked nipples are caused by other problems, such as a tongue tie. If adjustments to position and latching don't help, see if you can get a full oral assessment to check for tongue restriction. See the tongue tie chapter for more information about this.

Another cause of cracks and damage is a poorly fitting pump. We discuss flange sizing in the expressing chapter, and it really is important. If you're pumping and it's not comfortable, stop!

> *'I was in agony. Everyone kept telling me the latch was perfect, but I couldn't figure out how it could be if I was in so much pain and bleeding. I went to a support group and a breastfeeding counsellor helped me make some tiny changes to the way she latched and it was honestly like instant relief. They healed so quickly after that.'* – Fel, mum of Issy.

Treatments for cracked nipples

There are so many different lotions and potions on the market for cracked nipples. But the number one thing to remember in treating yourself is to find and sort the cause. No amount of special cream is going to help if there's a latch issue, for example.

The current recommendations for treating actual wounds and cracks in nipples, aside from correcting the problem, is moist wound healing. This means keeping the area moist, as it promotes faster healing (previously, we were told the exact opposite – to keep them as dry as possible and 'air them out'!).

What can you use to keep your nipple lubricated? Well, you've got something right at your fingertips: breastmilk! But if you want to use a product, you don't need to buy anything fancy. Good old petroleum jelly (branded products include Vaseline) has been found to be just as effective as the lanolin-based products that are popular. Anything a bit greasy will do, so, yep, a lanolin product can be fine, but a cheaper own brand one is all that's needed. Some recent research has confirmed coconut oil works well too.

You can also get other products, like gel pads, and gauze that is infused with paraffin, both of which aim to keep wounds moist and aid healing. These work in theory, but we don't have any evidence to back it up. They shouldn't be used over infections.

Silver nipple cups are one of the more expensive products on the market. These are a bit like a sort of flattened down thimble that you put over your nipple between feeds. The thought is that the silver, which to be fair people have used for a very long time for healing, will help. Whether it's that, or that there's no clothes or pads rubbing the nipple, or simply that the nipple might sit in a pool of your milk for a while, anecdotally lots of parents tell me they're effective. I haven't yet found any research to support their use, though, and some parents have reported they prevent healing, by keeping the damaged nipple too soggy.

Milk blisters/blebs

The nipple doesn't have just one hole/opening. In fact, most people have between ten and twenty on each nipple! But it can also be way more, or fewer. These openings can sometimes get blocked, or healed over with skin, and when it happens it can form a milk blister, or bleb. These can look like a small white or clear spot on the nipple, often just millimetres across. For something seemingly so small, they can cause a lot of pain and problems!

Described as a bruised feeling, extreme sensitivity, shooting pains (which can even go deep into the breast) or as very pinchy, most people certainly know something is wrong because of what they're feeling. Sometimes this pain comes on a day or two before the blister becomes apparent. Milk blisters are frequently misdiagnosed as thrush in my experience, or as a pus-filled spot, but they're very different. They are usually caused by nipple compression, where the nipple gets flattened during a feed and so the pore cannot empty properly and becomes blocked. Or they occur due to damage to the pore, that the body helpfully tries to heal by growing skin over it, which causes a blockage. Teething can also have an impact later down the line, mainly because the latch often changes. If not resolved, the milk can back up behind the blister, with potential for engorgement and mastitis.

As with a lot of breastfeeding difficulties, one of the key factors with blebs is resolving the underlying issue. So if the nipple is getting pinched by the latch, or the pump is the wrong fit, these things will need changing. It can also be really helpful to use moist heat over the nipple before each feed/expressing. A (comfortably) hot, wet flannel or muslin held over the nipple to soften the tissue should allow the milk to flow through more easily when you feed.

For persistent blebs, sometimes a mild steroid cream is prescribed to promote healing. Don't be tempted to pick at the blister, as this will just cause more inflammation and damage and prolong the problem and pain.

Very rarely, the blockage may need manually squeezing out, but definitely don't do this as a first port of call!

Vasospasm and Raynaud's

Vasospasm is when blood vessels very quickly contract, leaving blood flow restricted. This can feel very painful, and leaves the nipple blanched or paler in colour. For some people the pain is just in the nipple, others get shooting pain deep into the breast. This is usually caused, once again, by nipple compression coming from the latch, i.e. the nipple getting squished up against that hard palate in the mouth.

So the key, as ever, is often gonna be sorting that. Even if the vasospasm is caused by other issues, there are almost always adjustments to latch that will help too.

Other things that may cause vasospasms are cigarette smoking and caffeine. It's worth cutting these out, if you can. High levels of stress can also have an impact. Cold temperatures can trigger them too, so keeping your breasts/yourself warm is helpful. Putting something warm over the breast the minute your baby unlatches has been found to be very soothing for lots of parents. Keeping any breast pads/nipple creams/clothes tucked against your body to warm them whilst you feed is an easy way to manage this.

Never latch your baby (or pump) while you're having a vasospasm, as this will be very uncomfortable.

For some people, vasospasm may be part of another condition called Raynaud's. This is a disorder of the small blood vessels in the extremities (hands and feet), and it's relatively common. The hands and feet may feel very cold, painful or numb, and have colour changes such as paling of the skin or blue/purple in some skin tones. And it can happen with nipples too! It's distinguishable from vasospasms due to the effect the temperature has, and you're more likely to get a blue/purple colour change as well as blanching.

Alongside treatments you can do at home, which are the same as for vasospasms above, some people get treatment from their GP/care provider. A blood pressure medication called nifedipine has been found to be effective for some.

Unfortunately, your doctor may not have come across Raynaud's of the nipple, so if you think you may have this, perhaps ask for a referral to the infant feeding team for specialised support.

Infection

It's possible to get a bacterial infection in your nipple, especially if you've had cracks and damage. This can be really sore! If you've got damage and pain that is slow to heal despite the latch being bang on, it's well worth asking for a swab of your nipple to be taken, to check for infection (This is different to thrush, see more in chapter 7).

Skin conditions

You can get skin conditions such as eczema and psoriasis affecting your nipple and areola, and again these often get misdiagnosed as thrush. They can be incredibly uncomfortable.

If you already suffer with skin conditions, it may be that you have a better idea of what's going on, but if it's new to you, it can seem quite alarming sometimes.

Moisturisers and emollients can be prescribed/used, and occasionally steroid use may be needed. Please speak with your doctor.

If any of this is only showing up on one side, it's particularly important to get it looked at, as there is a rare form of breast cancer called Paget's disease that can look a lot like nipple eczema. Please don't panic, but do get checked out promptly.

Cream sensitivity

Interestingly, there have been quite a few occasions where clients of mine have been having nipple pain and damage, and once they've *stopped* using lotions, things have improved. A surprising amount of people are actually sensitive to the creams, especially lanolin. If you're using a product and things aren't improving, maybe stop using it and see what happens?

> 'When I was pregnant, everyone I knew said I had to get this particular cream. So I slapped it on and slapped it on. I had loads of pain and angry, flaky skin and everyone I saw kept making sure I was using cream to help. They even prescribed me thrush treatments, but they didn't work. Eventually, at about five weeks, someone advised me to stop the nipple cream and within two days it was completely better. I now know I have an allergy to lanolin.' – Anna, mum of Bhodi and Jack.

Menstrual cycle

Some people find that they get nipple pain when they're pre-menstrual and/or during the first few days of their period. When you get your period back varies massively, and while the average is when your baby is around fourteen months, it can happen as early as six weeks after birth (before then it's likely to still be bleeding related to the birth). So if feeding has been pain free and then you start to get unexplained tenderness on both sides, with no visible damage or pinching from latch, it could well be related to your periods.

What about nipple shields?

Ah, nipple shields. The marmite of the breastfeeding world! But why? Because nipple shields can make or break a breastfeeding journey, and I think that's why you hear such mixed opinions about them. Let's explore a bit.

Some people use shields when their baby can't latch at the breast for a reason such as flat or inverted nipples. The reason they work in this instance is because the sucking reflex is triggered when something hits the back of the roof of the baby's mouth, so the baby gets hold of the shield and sucking can start. For other people, a shield is used to help nipple pain or damage, as a sort of protective barrier.

Because babies come out with no preconceived notion of what a nipple will look like, it's definitely worth trying to latch the baby without shields for as long as you can, with lots of skin-to-skin time, as often they will manage without. It is perfectly possible in almost all cases for a baby to latch directly to the breast without causing damage and pain, so if you're considering using a shield for this reason, please seek support to see if some changes to the way baby latches can help instead. Get support with breast shaping, laid-back feeding and other techniques to help achieve a latch. And be sure to protect your milk supply and keep baby fed by hand expressing frequently.

For babies that just *can't* latch at the breast despite these measures, plus good support, time and patience, nipple shields can be absolutely amazing and keep breastfeeding going when it may otherwise have stopped.

So, let's assume from now on that you have chosen to use a shield. No matter the reason, there are things to consider. The first is that you will need to wait until you have larger quantities of milk (i.e., your milk 'comes in'), because colostrum, the sticky early milk, won't get transferred well with a shield.

The next is that some babies can't latch deeply enough to the breast with a shield in place. What this means is that there is a strong possibility the baby will not transfer as much milk as they need, and this leaves milk in your breasts, so your body thinks the milk is not needed and makes a bit less for the next day and the next day, and in the end milk supply will be impacted.

You might not notice this straight away, because, in the early days of breastfeeding, you often start with a bit of an oversupply of milk. So, in the short term, the baby may be able to get enough milk because of this. But it's really important to frequently assess that things are continuing to go well as milk supply settles. Remember: when under six weeks old, a baby should have six to eight or more heavy wet nappies a day, and do at least two poos. Of course, some people naturally have a tendency toward a bit of an oversupply in the long run, and, for those people, shields may not cause an issue, but for most people it does need to be closely monitored.

Another thing to consider with shields is that *sucking* at the breast does not necessarily mean *drinking* at the breast. Sadly, I have seen far too many parents battling to get baby to latch and then feeling so delighted to see baby sucking away happily, only to then find issues with weight and milk supply. Familiarise yourself with what it looks like when a baby is drinking and swallowing at the breast, and what a normal suck/swallow pattern for a baby looks like (see p. 58). This will really help you figure out if using shields is working for you.

Correctly applying the shield, and holding the baby in a way to encourage the deepest latch, are really important. Access skilled breastfeeding support for help with this.

So, for all of the above, this is why I say shields are love/hate. For some people using a shield can get a baby latching at the breast who otherwise wouldn't, and they carry on with no issues. For others, using a shield means their baby feeds very frequently and for a long time and still doesn't get enough milk.

I don't love *or* hate shields, personally; I'm very much in the 'if it helps you keep breastfeeding, I'm all for it' camp. But what I don't love is when parents haven't been given the full picture that there *can* be disadvantages to their use and it ends their breastfeeding journey earlier than they would have liked. And I'm definitely not a fan of a shield being given in place of good support!

How to apply a nipple shield

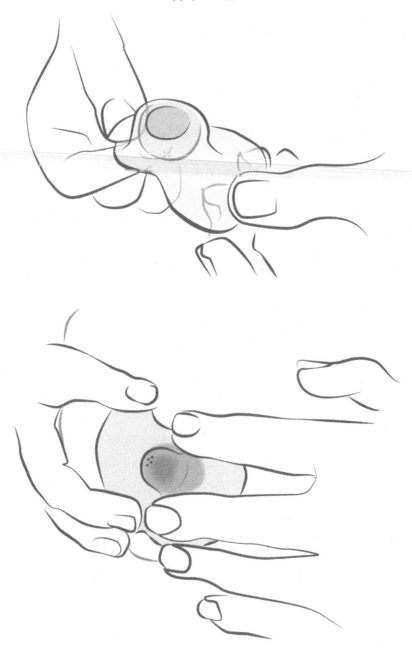

Positioning with a nipple shield

Position that may cause a shallow latch

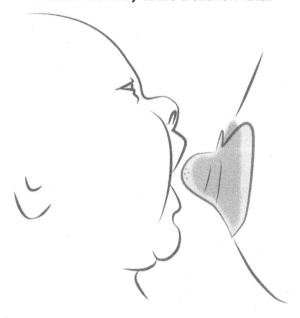

Position to help a deeper latch

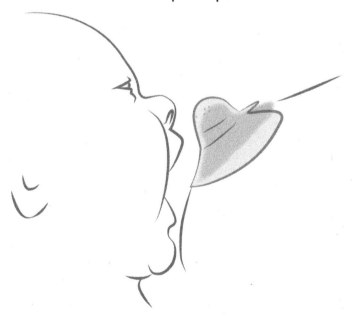

Conclusion

The most important thing I hope you get from this chapter is knowing that pain isn't normal. Temporary tenderness, maybe, but if it goes beyond that then it really is a sign that something isn't right or needs changing.

It can feel a bit like detective work figuring out what's causing problems sometimes – and that's for us as professionals – so please don't feel bad if you can't figure out the cause of your problem yourself.

Dealing with nipple pain and problems can be extremely hard, and can make you feel low and frustrated. Sometimes parents even have feelings of failing, which is a really horrible way to feel. Don't hesitate to get help if you're having any difficulties or worries at all. You're not alone.

Louise's story

I always wanted to breastfeed, and even before I got pregnant I knew this was the method of feeding I was always going to choose. There are obvious reasons why breastfeeding is more beneficial, and although those reasons did help me with my decision, breastfeeding was simply something I wanted, and it meant more than just a method of feeding.

I went to some breastfeeding workshops when I was pregnant with both of my boys, wanting to be prepared for when the time came.

My feeding journey with Charlie

Charlie was born via planned C-section due to being breech in January 2019. I was nervous for several reasons, but I had gone into theatre expressing that I ideally wanted skin to skin and to try feeding as soon as I could. But when Charlie was born, none of that was possible. He was born crying, but when they took him to do his checks, they were taking a little longer. I remember turning to Mike, worried, and asking if everything was okay. The doctors and midwives came over, explaining that he was having a little bit more trouble with his breathing; that they wanted to admit him to NICU so they could give him the help he needed. Obviously a scary moment, but I knew he was in the best hands.

I got to have a quick cuddle with him for a brief moment before he was whisked away in an incubator. At this point, feeding became the least of my worries. I headed back to recovery soon after and it felt like hours until I heard any updates on my baby boy. I was then taken down to the ward.

When I arrived, I do remember briefly a midwife asking how I wanted to feed and we discussed breastfeeding and hand expressing. She encouraged me to hand express every three hours, which I attempted, but had no success with. I also had no success after going up to NICU to see Charlie, so kept trying and trying to express. The next day, the NICU nurses asked if it was okay to give Charlie some formula, as he hadn't had any milk at this point, to which we both agreed, as he was on a feeding tube anyway and I just wasn't producing anything myself. I think that was the first time I felt some sort of guilt. Day Two was the first time we also had skin to skin and I could properly feel that bond.

I felt like Day Two was eventful: Charlie came out of the incubator and he got to wear clothes and then be discharged from NICU and put on the transition ward with me. I feel this is when our journey really began, and the days following were really an emotional rollercoaster that I try hard to forget.

It was late into the evening that Charlie was reunited with me. Mike was about to go home and I briefly had the midwives say that he would be due a feed with his feeding tube in x amount of hours, with no mention of me trying to feed or anything. I don't think I questioned it, as I was tired but also anxious. I remember an hour or so later pressing my buzzer and asking if he needed a feed through his tube, to which the midwife said I could try feeding him myself; she helped me latch him on and then left the room. He probably fed no longer than ten minutes before he unlatched and began to scream, so I then pressed my buzzer again. Next time, a nursery nurse came, I explained I was having trouble trying to latch him on and asked for help. So this is where she picked up Charlie, latched him on, made a comment along the lines of 'See, that was easy', and left the room. Of course, Charlie unlatched as soon as she left and began to scream again. I began to cry too. I honestly felt so vulnerable at that point; I was struggling to feed my child who was hungry, and I did not feel supported at all. I was too scared to ask for help again and tried and tried my best to settle him/latch him on. After about an hour of not having much luck, I gave in and walked to the desk and asked for some formula to feed him with. I was exhausted. I just didn't have it in me anymore to keep pushing for help and feeling ignored.

As the night went on, I walked down those corridors repeatedly asking for ready-made bottles of formula. I'd have hours with Charlie where he would just scream. I couldn't settle him, I couldn't latch him and, despite my efforts, I was just having no luck, and the midwives were not interested. I just felt like a huge failure. I remember, the next morning, Mike coming in for the day; I told him all about the night and asked if he could stay the next night with me (it was pre-Covid, so it was allowed), as I needed him to be my voice while I was not in a fit state to be able to raise mine.

The next two nights were slightly better. I had some really helpful midwives and MCAs on the night shift who helped me with feeding positions and cup feeding also. They would sit with me to make sure I was comfortable with what I was doing. They were a huge help and, for the first time in hospital, I began to believe I could actually do this.

I was discharged after a four-night stay feeling a little nervous about it all, but like I was in a better place to give it a good go.

The first night was hell, probably on par with my first night alone with Charlie in the hospital, maybe a little worse, because I didn't have a buzzer by my side – this was the real thing, and I just couldn't do it. I tried to feed, I practised all the positions we had done in hospital, but he just wouldn't stay latched on long enough. I actually remember sitting on the edge of the bed, holding Charlie in my arms, tears running down my face, Charlie screaming and me rocking back and forwards, just repeating the words 'I can't do this'.

The next day, my community midwife came to visit. We discussed feeding, where I admitted I was really struggling and that my mental health was at an all-time low. I decided I needed time to think about this so I made the decision to express, formula feed and keep attempting to put Charlie on the breast at the times it wasn't driving me to rock bottom. The midwife said it was my choice, and if I wanted to do that then that was fine.

I continued to express for thirteen weeks, but not exclusively or anything. I could probably only express enough to make one bottle of breastmilk in a space of four days or so, but it was what kept me going. After those thirteen weeks, my milk supply significantly dropped and I had to plead with myself to stop. It was a horrible decision to make and I cried hopelessly for weeks to follow. It completely broke me: this wasn't the choice I wanted to make yet the only one I could.

Charlie was thriving on formula, but I was grieving, grieving the journey I never had. And then, just as I was starting to accept what had happened, Charlie's six-month check came about and the health visitor said, 'It looks like he has tongue tie', and after a further look, she said she was 99.9 per cent sure it was tongue tie. I was gutted, and questioned how that got missed, after all the checks he had in hospital, after all the cries for help, after everything I had been through, *this* is what I find out. I was so angry and felt so let down.

I struggled with this for months, actually. I spoke about it in some CBT, and I remember my therapist really focusing on reminding me that I did not *fail*, and that instead I was *failed*. No matter how much I tried, it was physically difficult for me to feed, and there was nothing I could have done differently. I often remind myself of this.

I will always hold on to the memories I had feeding Charlie – the good, the bad, the hard times – because it was a huge part of my journey with him, but I knew that when I had another baby, I would push hard for the support that I never had with Charlie, and I would have the breastfeeding journey that I'd always wanted; I just felt a little sad it wouldn't be with him.

My feeding journey with Hugo

This part is a lot less depressing, I promise. Don't get me wrong: I still had my struggles, it has still been an emotional journey, but I suppose I can say I've got my happy ending, finally.

When I fell pregnant with Hugo, I was determined to breastfeed. In fact, I gave myself no other option. I'm not sure if it was a good thing that I didn't allow myself a backup or if I was potentially setting myself up for disappointment. But I told myself, and everyone else for that matter, that I *would* breastfeed and that was that. I attended breastfeeding workshops, spoke to others and did my research, so that I could stay determined and also have the knowledge for when it came to it.

89

The first challenge I was hit with was that I was diagnosed with gestational diabetes in pregnancy, and soon became aware how important it was for the baby to have breastmilk to help with his blood sugar when he was born. My diabetic team advised it would be beneficial for me to collect colostrum in a syringe from 36 weeks, which could help if we were faced with any feeding difficulties when he was born. I hadn't heard of this when I had Charlie. This was something I definitely wanted to try, so, at my 36-week appointment, I was given a pack for this. I managed to hand express just under 1ml a day and, by the time, I went in for my second C-section, I had collected about fifteen syringes. I felt so confident about feeding at this point.

I went into hospital on 1 July to have my elective caesarean. Ironically, the same morning my waters broke, and Hugo was born at 9:57am. He came out with a huge set of lungs on him! He was perfect and I got to have skin to skin with him as soon as he was cleaned up. He was mine and I had him in my arms the whole time; completely different to what I had experienced with Charlie.

I went back to recovery and, shortly after Hugo was born, I got to feed him. He latched on and I couldn't believe it; I was feeding him by myself without the help of anyone else. It felt magical, it really did. He also passed his first blood-sugar reading with flying colours and I felt way more confident with feeding as the hours went on.

Day Two down on the ward, I had a visit from the infant feeding team, who although they weren't concerned, helped me get a deeper latch with Hugo and also made sure he wasn't getting too tired when on the breast, so helped me with that too. We had arranged for the infant feeding team to do a home visit as well.

Louise's story

We are now just over six months into my feeding journey and I have never been prouder of myself. It took so long to get here, so many challenges. It's been a huge rollercoaster, but I've got this far and I don't plan to stop any time soon.

6

Weight gain and milk supply

'How much did she weigh?!'

Often one of the very first questions you're asked by friends and family when your baby arrives is about the weight. Weight checks can play a big part in assessing your baby's growth and health, but also how things are going with feeding. But it's *not* the whole picture! Weight measurements shouldn't be used as the sole piece of information for figuring out how feeding is going, as there are lots of other factors to take into consideration.

Anyone weighing your baby should be able to help you interpret the measurements and what they mean for your own individual situation, but I'll break it down for you here so that you've got a good idea of what's normal, and what might be suggested if they're not gaining weight as expected. Remember that this is *your* baby and *your* feeding journey. You should be given information, options and possibly recommendations, but it's not up to anyone else what you do. It's for you to make the final decisions. If you feel uncomfortable with any suggestions, get a second opinion.

The first few days

In the beginning, babies often lose some weight initially, and this can be normal as long as it's not excessive and everything else is going well. They're usually weighed again when they are three or five days old, depending on your local maternity guidelines.

A weight loss of up to 7–8 per cent of the birthweight is generally considered fine. Though, if you have any feeding problems (pain, latching difficulties or anything else), these shouldn't be ignored just because weight loss is okay.

A weight loss of 10 per cent or above should mean a skilled person sits with you, supporting you through a full feed, and leaves you with a plan that hopefully helps you move forward. And above 12–12.5 per cent usually means a medical review as well as the above, and often readmission to hospital too, to make sure you're well supported.

After the first weight check

From the point of the initial 3-to-5-day weight check with that possible loss, babies should gain weight at every check from there on. No further weight loss is expected. Don't get me wrong: further weight loss does happen sometimes, but it usually means something's been going on with the feeding rather than it being an expected occurrence. Usually, all being well, they will be back to their birth weight by or before they're two weeks old.

Babies will gain 30–40g a day (7–10 ounces a week) on average in the first three months, and weights will usually be plotted on a centile chart (see below). They should be weighed at least weekly until feeding feels established and they are growing reliably. But they should be weighed no more frequently than monthly thereafter.

Centile charts

Centile charts look a little like a graph, and are a place for your baby's weight and age to be plotted. This will then tell you which 'centile' they are on or around. We are not aiming for them to be on any particular centile, per se, as every baby is different, but for them to remain fairly consistently on the same one, more or less.

These centile lines are a percentage marker. So, if your baby is on the 50th percentile, bang in the middle of the chart, that means 50 per cent of babies will be bigger, and 50 per cent will be smaller. If they're on the 98th centile, 2 per cent of babies are bigger, 98 per cent are smaller. If they're on the 2nd centile, 2 per cent are smaller, 98 per cent are bigger. And so on.

As I said, it's absolutely okay to be a bigger or smaller baby – we're all different, after all – but it's important that they follow that line roughly, as that's what shows us they're growing appropriately and consistently.

Faltering growth

If a baby is not gaining weight as expected, and moving down across the centile lines rather than following them, this needs investigating, and feeding (and possibly medical) support should be accessed promptly.

'Are they not just finding their own line?' This is something that parents have previously been told, but it's very rarely the case.

There are thresholds that can help you figure out if your baby's chart is of concern.

Weight thresholds

If your baby isn't back to birth weight by Week 3.

A fall across one or more centiles if your baby was born on the 9th centile or below.

A fall across two or more centiles if they were born between the 9th and 91st centile.

A fall across three or more centiles if they were born above the 91st centile.

If they fall below the second centile no matter what they were born on.

Ideally, though, don't wait until it gets to this point to access support. If you can see the trajectory of your baby's weight is heading down across the centiles, get a feeding assessment with a trained professional. It's much easier to make changes sooner rather than later. Just reweighing, watching and waiting is unlikely to be helpful or change anything.

Why aren't they gaining weight?

There are a lot of potential reasons for babies not to gain weight as expected, and an experienced professional will be able to assess your situation and help you figure out what's going on. Overwhelmingly, though, the main cause is because they need more milk. This may be because they're not feeding often enough, not feeding effectively enough, or because there's a problem with supply. These things can all overlap, of course, and it's common that if a baby isn't feeding effectively for supply to drop (remember: the more milk they remove – the more you make, so if they're not removing enough milk, you won't make enough milk). In most cases this can be sorted, however, so please don't feel you have to stop breastfeeding!

What can I do to help them gain weight/increase my supply?

There are some key things you can do if your baby isn't gaining weight well that can be hugely effective.

- **Go back to basics with positioning and latch**. This is so important and has an enormous impact on their ability to transfer (move and drink) milk and, in turn, your supply.

  Even if you've been told your latch looks great, there are almost always changes that can be made to make things more effective.

- **Feed frequently**. At *least* eight times every 24 hours, but twelve or more may be more realistic.

- **Breast compressions**. This is a technique you can use to help move a little more milk into the baby, or even cause another milk ejection. Using your hand, you cup any part of your breast you can get to, fairly far back toward the chest wall so that you don't dislodge the latch. When the baby is sucking, you firmly but comfortably squeeze your breast, and hold that squeeze until the baby takes a pause in sucking, then you release. If you notice the baby swallows more doing this, continue to use the same technique in the same spot. If they don't swallow more, try moving your hand around slightly to a different spot and try again.

– **Use both breasts at each feed, maybe even more than once**. We're often told to keep the baby on the same breast to ensure they get 'the fatty milk' (see p. 211), but, in reality, it's the total volume of milk taken in 24 hours that determines weight gain. Swapping sides, or 'switch feeding', encourages another milk ejection, which in turn encourages the baby to drink more, gain weight better and increase your supply to boot! So please do switch sides during a feed; you can even do it multiple times. Watch for your baby's active feeding to decrease and swallowing to slow down and stop, as this is the sign to switch sides (perhaps after trying some compressions first).

– **Familiarise yourself with your baby's sucking pattern and encourage as much 'active' feeding as you can**. The part when they're alert and sucking well with lots of swallows is the bit we want plenty of. A baby that is sleepily sucking and not swallowing much won't be taking much milk. Encourage active feeding by using compressions, switching sides frequently, skin contact, and nappy changes between boobs.

– **Call in your helpers**. When your baby is having weight difficulties, it can be quite stressful and worrying. It can also be quite time consuming doing the things you need to do to make things improve. So now is a really good time to reach out to your support network. Can they cook you some meals for the freezer? Could they do some laundry or your hoovering? Even just some company is beneficial. People love to help on the whole, especially where babies are involved, so don't be afraid to reach out.

– **Get specialist support.** If you can access an IBCLC, then do it.

Do I need teas/supplements/cookies for my milk supply?

There are lots of products on the market that claim to help support or increase milk supply. In reality, we just don't have the research to back this up at all.

There is even a pack of special lactation cookies in my local supermarket that cost more than this book for just one pack! But what you eat, drink or take doesn't have an impact on your supply, so avoid! Hey, if someone wants to make you some nice cookies or flapjacks with ingredients in them that are said to help supply, don't turn them down, because, frankly, nice treats can do us good mentally, and being looked after can be really beneficial for milk supply. And if someone has got you some tea and you like it, drink it, sure, but please don't feel you have to force yourself to, as it's very unlikely to make any difference.

Truly, if I could tell you that eating or drinking something would make a change and make things easier, I would.

Feeding plans

On top of everything I've outlined above, sometimes you may be encouraged to go onto a 'feeding plan'. These can be really effective at increasing milk supply and/or baby's weight, but they can be pretty challenging, too.

An example would be where you're told to feed the baby, then express milk, then offer the baby that expressed milk too, and do this three hourly, all day and night. You might hear this called Triple Feeding. As you can imagine, this barely leaves any room to do anything else, so eating and sleeping (though vital) are almost impossible.

There are ways to make it easier, though, which I'll outline here.

Firstly, make sure you've addressed everything I've outlined above: a deep asymmetric latch, you're watching for active feeding (the bit where you really notice your baby swallowing – if you're not sure, *do* get someone skilled to notice your baby's swallows with you) and encouraging your supply by using breast compressions and switch feeding. It may be that limiting the feed to 20 or 30 minutes of this might be useful – it may seem counterproductive taking your baby *off* the breast, but if they are not effectively feeding at this point, then it's better to move on to the next stage of the plan and make it as time efficient as possible.

'Why can't I just let the baby feed for longer?' For most people in the situation of needing this feeding plan, the baby isn't feeding as effectively as is needed to get enough milk or maintain supply. So, to continue letting the baby just feed with really infrequent swallows is unlikely to change anything, and may even make things worse. Expressing as the next stage is a way of ensuring your breasts get additional effective stimulation, and some extra milk to give to the baby that they may not have managed to get themselves (at the moment).

Secondly, how you express can make a big difference. Check out the chapter on expressing for tips on how to make this as effective as possible. Key points to remember, though, are to get comfy, with lots of gentle breast massage before and during pumping; to use a combo of hand expressing and pumping (use a hospital grade double pump where possible, and check the pump is the right fit for you). The recommended frequency to express is six to eight times each 24 hours, including at least once at night (between 1 and 5am, ideally). In reality, it can be extremely difficult to fit this amount in and can cause a lot of stress, which in turn isn't helpful with milk flow and relaxed feeding. Do what you can, and remember that frequency is likely to be more important than the amount of time spent. So it's better to do six lots of 5 minutes than one session of 30 minutes.

Lastly, let's look at giving additional milk, also known as supplementing or 'topping up'. This last part of the feeding plan is giving the baby the additional milk you've expressed, and/or sometimes some formula, if the expressed milk amounts are not yet enough. The amounts recommended for top-ups vary depending on the age of the baby, how effectively they're feeding, and what's been happening with their growth and nappy output. As a rough guide, though, they will usually be around 15–45ml (0.5 to 1.5 ounces) per feed, given three-hourly as a maximum. Any more than that isn't a top up, more a replacement of a full feed. A calculation will often be used to help work out how much extra milk to give. This is usually based on 150ml per kilo of your baby's weight per day.

As a starting point, you may give half or a quarter of that over 24 hours, and see how weight gain goes. For example, if your baby weighs 4kg, you would give them 4 x 150ml, which equals 600ml. But 600ml would be a lot to give in a day straight away, so reducing the amount may make sense to start with. Half of 600ml is 300, and if we divide that by eight feeds, that's 37.5ml given around every three hours.

Three-hourly top-ups are not a hard and fast rule, though, and if it's easier or suits you better to give that over four or six feeds, that's fine. We ideally don't want to give this amount over two or three feeds, however, as this would mean quite large volumes for a baby to take in.

The idea is that we want to give the baby enough extra milk that they gain weight and have enough energy to feed more effectively, but we don't want to give them so much that they don't want to go to the breast frequently. We also don't want to stretch their tummy and make them uncomfortable by giving them large volumes, which could mean they're less settled at the breast later on.

How to give the top-up milk

There are lots of ways you can give top-up milk, and there are pros and cons to each. If you feel overwhelmed by the choice, that's understandable and absolutely okay; find out more about them and trust your instinct on what feels the right choice for you.

The most common approach, of course, is to use a bottle. The good thing about this is that it's easily accessible and something most people feel comfortable using. The difficulties can be that the milk can be fed very quickly to the baby, which can make them uncomfortable and gassy, and they may not recognise that the feed has finished. There is also a school of thought that feeding from a bottle teat can cause problems with the way they latch and feed at the breast, sometimes called 'nipple confusion'. Sometimes they can find the bottle easier to feed from if the flow is fast, you see, and this may even lead to a bottle preference and refusal and rejection of the breast, which, as I'm sure you can imagine, can be really upsetting.

The key to minimising these difficulties is to use a technique called paced feeding. See the chapter on expressing for more information about how to do this.

Cup feeding is another method of giving top ups that's been used for many years. It can avoid the possible nipple confusion problem, but can be trickier to do and milk can easily be spilled and wasted – difficult to be complacent about when your expressed milk is so precious! There is evidence that cup feeding exercises similar muscles used in breast feeding, much more than with bottle feeding, so this in itself may be an advantage. It's not suitable for babies that are very sleepy, though, as there is a risk of breathing in the milk rather than drinking it.

Syringe feeding (minus the needle, of course) is when you pop a breastfeeding syringe in the corner of the baby's mouth and very slowly and gradually push in tiny amounts of milk and let them swallow it down. This can be good for small amounts of milk, but isn't really practical for higher volumes. Syringe feeding is not a long-term solution, so if you've been doing it for more than a few days, talk to your midwife.

Supplementing via tube during a breastfeed is yet another approach. And, I won't lie: this is my favourite method! It can be a little bit faffy to get started, but once you've practised a bit, it can be a game changer. You can either get hold of specific equipment known as a supplementary nursing system (SNS) made to do this, or you can make a homemade version using a feeding tube – the type of tube used in hospitals that go up someone's nose into their tummy. Know the ones? But you don't put it up your baby's nose. Instead you use it a bit like a baby straw. One end of the tube goes into a bottle of milk that you're giving, the other slips into the corner of their mouth whilst they breastfeed. When they suck at the breast, they also get small amounts of the top up milk at the same time.

What I like about this is that not only does it cut down on time, but also gives extra breast stimulation, along with positive association with breastfeeding and reducing possible teat confusion too. That's not to say it's all pros, though, as some people really do find it too faffy and off putting, and occasionally some babies prefer the faster flow with the tube in place and can reject the breast without.

Supplementing via a tube may not be a method that will be discussed with you as standard, but it's well worth having a think about, especially if you are likely to be giving additional milk for more than a couple of days. Your local infant feeding team or an IBCLC should be able to help you with this if you need it.

> 'I'd been having problems with my baby's weight gain for a while, and had been on a triple feeding plan for what felt like for ever. I'd been feeding, expressing, and topping up by bottle. It was a lot. My baby was getting fussier at the breast and enjoying the bottle more and more; it was breaking my heart, to be honest.

'*Someone suggested I try the "tube and boob", and I tried it as a bit of a last resort before I quit breastfeeding. Well, it absolutely saved us, no doubt in my mind.*

'*It was definitely difficult to get started, and I almost didn't bother, but something in me was so desperate to keep going that I kept trying. Once I'd managed it, it was so fantastic to see him drinking the top-up milk she needed while breastfeeding. It meant we were able to carry on breastfeeding for much longer and I'm so glad of that.*' – Bec, mum to Anabel.

What if the feeding plan isn't working?

If your baby's nappy output doesn't improve, or their weight gain doesn't increase enough, the first thing to do (alongside medical review) is to revisit all the basics again. So going back to latch, are you using compressions, are you feeding frequently enough (at least eight feeds each 24 hours), is there room to squeeze in an extra feed? Are you switching sides (or have you been told to stay on the same side – see the myths chapter about this). Are you managing to express? Is your pump the right fit for you? Could you manage to squeeze in an extra pumping session? Could you do a power pumping session (see below)?

Once you've revisited everything, and you feel everything is as good as you can get it, it may be worth considering if the top-up volumes are correct. Does your baby need some more supplemental milk?

I know giving more top-up milk can feel like a backward step and may be really disheartening, but making sure the baby is growing and well is paramount, and it is also actually a positive step towards breastfeeding going well. As babies get more energy and strength, they often breastfeed more effectively, which in turn leads to boosted supply, and so the upward spiral continues.

Having the baby medically reviewed is also important, because we want to make sure the reason for the weight difficulty isn't an underlying medical reason.

Power pumping

A power pumping session aims to mimic a baby's cluster feeding and can be a powerful supply booster. It replaces one pumping session, and is done over an hour. A correctly fitting double hospital-grade pump is ideal for this, if possible.

You start with some breast massage and hand expressing.

Pump for 20 mins

Rest for 10 mins

Pump for 10 mins

Rest for 10 mins

Pump for 10 mins

End with hand expressing.

How do I stop giving top ups?

It's not uncommon to feel like you've been put on a feeding plan, or told to top up, but not told how or when to stop following the plan and topping up.

The first thing to consider is if your little one is now growing well and consistently. If you drop top ups too soon, it can set you back and make things even harder.

Continue carrying on with them until you've had several weight checks that are an improvement, and also established that your baby's nappy output is as expected for their age or has increased. Once this is the case, it's worth dropping them down slowly, to allow your baby, and your body, to adjust to the change.

One method I suggest for this is to drop 30mls off the 24 hour total every few days or so. For example, if you're giving 400ml in top ups over 24 hours, drop it down to 370ml for several days. If you feel things are okay at that point, consider dropping down to 340ml for several days. Remember to keep going with the basics, and know that your little one may want to feed a bit more, and that that is normal and to be expected.

Continue to get your baby weighed at least weekly while you reduce the top ups, and if at any point things aren't as expected, don't drop down any further, and consider temporarily increasing again until you can get some support for moving forward.

'Every time I knew I was seeing the health visitor, I'd get filled with dread wondering what the scales would say. We'd weigh him and she'd plot his weight and it would have dropped down the lines a little further. She'd show me where it was and say I needed to come back next week to check again. But every time, she wasn't happy with it and just kept telling me to come back again. Eventually I asked for a referral to the infant feeding team and they helped me make some changes to the way he was feeding and put us on a feeding plan. It was really hard work, but it did make a difference. I just wish someone had done something sooner and not just kept rechecking every week.' – Anna, mum of Hamish.

Emotions

I won't lie: you may well feel a lot of emotions during this time. It can be extremely hard to be in this situation. Helpful friends and family may try to encourage you to move to formula feeding to save yourself these difficulties, but, in my experience, this is rarely what parents want to do. We have a culture of offering a formula solution to breastfeeding problems; it always comes from a well-meaning place, but it can feel demoralising. Try to be honest with them about what you want and need, and how they can best support you.

It's okay to find this hard; it's okay to feel sad about it, and worried, but that doesn't mean you want to stop! Please, above all, try to be kind to yourself while you're going through this. You *will* come out the other side, but for now it can be a struggle and you're bound to feel up and down.

If you can't make enough milk long term

For some people, sadly, they really can't make enough milk, no matter what they do. We don't really know how many people can't make enough milk, but in my experience it is a very small percentage. Unfortunately, before arriving at this conclusion they've often worked really hard and invested a lot of time, energy and emotion into feeding their baby. To then find they can't fully breastfeed can be extremely upsetting, and parents often report feelings much like grief.

Some of the more likely reasons for long term milk supply difficulties are hormonal issues and insufficient glandular tissue. Polycystic ovary syndrome (PCOS) or diabetes are two examples of hormonal issues that can impact on milk making. That's not to say that, if you have one of these conditions, you'll definitely have difficulties, so please don't worry unnecessarily. There are many parents with these issues that breastfeed with no problems with supply. If you're having problems with milk supply and know you have these conditions, it's well worth working with an IBCLC.

Insufficient glandular tissues (IGT) is where milk-making tissue in the breast hasn't developed as it might, and it means the amount of milk you can make is limited. Parents are often aware there was something different about their breasts before they had a baby. Signs of IGT can be:

- Widely spaced breasts.

- Long tubular breasts.

- Bulbous areola.

- A marked difference between your two breasts.

- No breast changes during pregnancy.

- No breast changes/fullness in the first week after birth.

Speak with your health-care provider if you feel any of this applies to you and you're having supply issues.

In situations where milk supply is limited, it can be incredibly emotional and hard. You can feel like you've failed. You can feel judged. You can feel resentful. It may feel so unfair when you so desperately want to feed your baby and have to also use donor milk or formula. If this is you: it's not what you wanted, I know, and it really hurts. Know that whatever you're feeling is absolutely okay, that your feelings are completely valid.

A lot of parents can find enormous comfort in the knowledge that breastfeeding is about much more than just providing milk. It can provide comfort, support sleep, and create a close bond, to name just a few benefits. Even those with a very low supply can still breastfeed and get great pleasure from it. Work with an IBCLC to help maximise breastfeeding, but also to help you with your thoughts and feelings about feeding your baby.

> '*After a long battle to conceive, I had my heart set on exclusively breastfeeding; it just meant so much to me. Unfortunately, with PCOS and IGT, exclusively breastfeeding wasn't going to happen and it took me a long time to come to terms with that. I felt inadequate, like I wasn't fulfilling my role as a mother, and at first I thought I was going to have to stop as I didn't realise I could combination feed long term. It just wasn't talked about as an option! I was met with dismissive comments from well-meaning friends and family who just didn't understand how important it was to me, but, thankfully, I found a support network who really drove me forward and educated me. I wanted to protect breastfeeding as much as possible, so we ensured we paced our bottle feeds and used an at-the-breast supplementary nursing system in the early months, which was a little faffy but great to get formula into my baby as well as stimulating my supply. For me, it wasn't a long-term solution, but once I was happy that breastfeeding was well established, I stopped using it. I continued to breastfeed my daughter until she was almost three-and-a-half years old.*' – Gemma, mum to Dotty and Josie.

Conclusion

Weight gain challenges, milk supply challenges, or both, can be an extremely difficult situation and test you to your limits. If it's happening to you, firstly, I'm really sorry – I know it's so tough. I really hope you've found the information in this chapter useful for moving forward, and I'd encourage you to work with an IBCLC if you possibly can.

Julia's story

I'm not one for routine, or being organised, so the thought of sterilising bottles, and strict time schedules for feeding, terrified me. Breastfeeding just made sense. No equipment, no feeding time slots. Perfect. It never crossed my mind that I wouldn't be able to do it, or that it might be difficult. Two days in it was clear: it wasn't easy, and it was going to be difficult. Very difficult! My son didn't seem to want to latch; it was like he didn't know what to do. He just threw his head round a lot, and kept spitting my nipple out. Five days after birth, still in hospital, my son was dropping weight as I desperately tried to feed him often with a tiny spoon or syringe. Different helpful midwives manhandling my boobs – 'try this, try that' – was not how I imagined it. After gaining enough weight, I was allowed home, but things didn't improve, and I was calling my best friend (a breastfeeding counsellor) at all sorts of hours . . . She would calmly sort me out, taking me through the different techniques and ideas, until he would latch and have a beautiful long feed. Until the next time . . . I soon realised I couldn't call her every time he was hungry (although I probably did the first week).

I wasn't going to give up, though. The thought of panicking to find a shop at 3am because we had run out of formula was enough motivation for me, but I could now see why people give up by this point. I had a specialist on speed dial, and yet I was struggling. How hard would it be for others?

Eventually, after about a month of perfecting techniques, perseverance, quite a few tears, and lots of my best friend's time, I was finally able to settle in a unscheduled routine of sitting on the sofa binge-eating chocolate and watching Netflix with a content feeding baby. Definitely worth it in the long run. Yes, there was lots of missed sleep, lots of eating one handed in restaurants while my husband chopped my pizza up for me, but I got used to it . . . I also got the best bits of 'Sorry, can you cook the tea? Baby needs feeding' or texting 'I'm going to be late – I'm still feeding' (while I paused Netflix).

Once I knew what I was doing, I also had this lack of stress that I saw other mums now experiencing – all that 'Why is he hungry? He has just fed!' or 'Why isn't he hungry? His bottle is overdue'. They had ditched their 'I can't breastfeed stress' in the early weeks, and replaced it with struggling to keep to unpredictable bottle-feeding routines and schedules. I was now past my stress and enjoying my lack of it. Once I got my head around the idea that baby will feed and sleep when it wants to, I just got on with it. One year and four months (and lots of box sets) later, I was sad to see it come to an end, but I definitely believe it was worth those first few tough months.

7

Breast pain and problems

'I was so worried about getting mastitis, but I've managed to avoid it so far. I learned all I could about how to prevent it and I think that really helped' – Camilla, mum of Leo.

During the time you're breastfeeding, you may experience lots of changes in your breasts, including growth, colour changes, visible veins for some skin tones, and more. But pain, on the whole, is not something normal. There are times when discomfort is more likely, but at other times it's a real red flag that problems are happening. So I thought we'd have a look in this chapter at some of the things that can cause pain, and at some breast problems that can happen for some people. Please try not to let it worry you, though, because, actually, a lot of these things are preventable, and certainly treatable.

Let's go . . .

Engorgement

Breasts that are very full of milk, swollen, or both, are referred to as engorged. This can be very painful, and can cause milk flow to slow down if severe.

A reasonable number of parents experience some engorgement in the early days when their breasts start to produce larger volumes of milk quite rapidly (often known as the milk 'coming in', which usually happens around Day 3–5). While it's common in the beginning, it's not something to just assume is normal and put up with. It could be a sign that your breasts aren't being drained effectively during feeds (due to position or latch issues), or that your baby isn't feeding frequently enough, for example.

'My boobs were like boulders stuck on my front. I thought it was normal because everyone had said I'd have a day where I looked like I'd had a bad boob job. They were tight and shiny and painful and it was making me feel quite upset.

Luckily, the midwife came that day and we changed how Ruby was feeding and things got better really quickly' – Billie, mum of Ruby.

Engorgement after the first week or so is not expected, and is a sign that something isn't quite right. Causes include the way the baby is feeding, infrequent feeding, a poor-fitting bra, using a nipple shield, or having too much milk. Self-help measures are the same as above, but, also, do try to speak to a feeding specialist to figure out the cause and improve things. Once you've double checked that, there are some other things you can do in these first few days.

Reverse pressure softening

Sometimes it can be difficult to latch the baby if around the nipple and areola is very hard with milk and swelling. To help with this, you can use a technique called reverse pressure softening. You use your fingers to gently but firmly push the breast backward steadily towards your chest and hold there for around 30 to 60 seconds. Your fingers should be placed at the base of your nipple on your areola and breast around it. Doing this lying

Reverse pressure softening

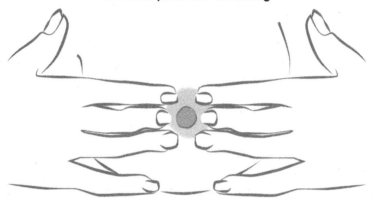

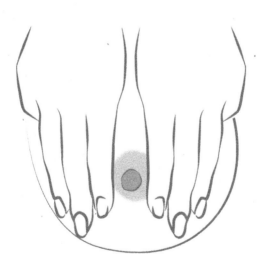

on your back can be helpful, and it should be done just before getting the baby to latch, as the area will often refill quite quickly.

Warmth and cold

Warm compresses can feel very soothing, and some parents find it helps milk to flow, which can relieve fullness and discomfort. However, for some people the heat can increase inflammation. Cool compresses can help with this.

Feed frequently

It is really important to feed often when you're engorged, even though you may not feel like it. Skipping feeds or stretching out the gap between feeds will make your breasts even fuller, which can make latching extra tricky, and sometimes lead to a cascade of problems, even mastitis (more on this in a later chapter). The best way to avoid engorgement and complications is to feed really frequently when you feel your milk coming in. It's fine to wake your baby to feed if you need them to: you're a team.

Pain killers

Pain killers are there if you need them. As long as you're not allergic or intolerant to them in any way, we know that there are a lot of simple painkillers, like paracetamol and ibuprofen, that can be hugely effective and are compatible with breastfeeding.

Blocked ducts

There are different theories as to what causes a 'blocked duct', from a thickening of milk blocking the way, to inflammation around the duct causing it to narrow, or even bacterial issues. What we do know is that the milk sometimes cannot flow from one area of the breast for some reason. This causes a firm or hard lump or wedge shape to form, that's usually a bruised feeling or painful. This can compress other areas in the breast, leading to more areas getting engorged or blocked and possibly leading to mastitis (see below), so it's not something to ignore.

Blocked ducts can be caused by a multitude of different things. I expect you may be able to guess by now what I'm going to say . . . check your latch! The way the baby is latched at the breast affects how the milk is drained. If it's not drained properly, this can lead to blocked ducts. If a feed is missed or skipped, this can cause a blocked duct too, as can wearing bras or clothing that compress an area of your breast. Basically, anything that could potentially stop milk from flowing has the potential to cause blocked ducts and inflamed areas in the breast.

It's a good idea to feel your breasts after feeds a couple of times a day, and just get used to what they feel like after your baby has had a really good feed. Being confident in what they normally feel like helps you notice any blocked ducts early and makes it easier to get things moving again. If you notice any lumps or bumps that you don't think are blocked ducts, and don't go after a good feed, do see your GP. There are lots of lumps and bumps in breasts that are not the scary ones, though, so please don't worry, but do get checked nevertheless.

It can be hard to try and decide whether it's a blocked duct or mastitis at times, but luckily a lot of the treatment is the same. If in doubt, reach out.

Mastitis

A lot of people have heard of mastitis, and most people seem to think of it as a breast infection requiring antibiotics, which is what we traditionally thought. But information has recently changed, so I'll outline it here.

Mastitis is inflammation of the breast, usually one area, but sometimes the whole breast. Typically, milk doesn't flow well because of this inflammation, making things worse. It can be very painful, and the breast will often be hard, hot, and redness will be seen on some skin tones. Mastitis can give you flu-like symptoms and a temperature.

All mastitis cases will benefit from measures to reduce inflammation. Some mastitis cases will need antibiotics if there is also infection. The guidance is to use self-help measures, and seek medical advice if symptoms don't improve within 12–24 hours, or if they worsen quickly.

Self-help measures for mastitis

If you suspect you have mastitis, feed as normal; don't add in any extra feeds, as you don't want to increase milk supply, which would exacerbate the problem. Similarly, avoid breast pump use or expressing if this isn't something you usually do.

We used to advise lots of massage, and people even recommended using electric toothbrushes to vigorously massage the breast, but this is really not helpful! Deep massage like this can cause inflammation to increase, stop things improving and even make things worse.

Light-touch massage, to encourage lymph drainage, may be beneficial, however. This involves stroking from the nipple towards the armpit. The aim is to reduce the extra fluid (causing swelling and pressure) in the breast tissue and move it through the body's natural drainage system.

Over the counter anti-inflammatory medications, such as ibuprofen, can help with pain but also decrease swelling. Follow the instructions as per the packet, and speak to a health professional if you have any queries or concerns.

Cool or cold compresses can also be used to relieve symptoms, as it will reduce the extra fluid and inflammation and can be soothing by itself. Some parents find warmth may help with the discomfort, but it may, in theory, make the inflammation a little worse. So use with caution – listen to your body.

When you have mastitis, it's important that you look after yourself a bit like if you had flu. So bed rest and lots of fluids, and other people looking after the kids and house! Don't put on a brave face.

Antibiotics?

Some cases of mastitis are caused by bacterial infection and require antibiotics. Because it can be hard to tell which mastitis cases require antibiotics, doctors tend to prescribe them to be on the safe side. This is something you can discuss with them at your appointment, and the Academy of Breastfeeding Medicine has a protocol for health professionals which it may be useful to direct your doctor to.

Breast abscess

A breast abscess is a lump that is actually a collection of pus (Yuck! Sorry!). They happen most commonly if mastitis isn't treated correctly, for example if you were told to stop or restrict breastfeeding during a bout of mastitis. Sometimes you can feel them, sometimes you can see them. They can be painful, and symptoms can feel similar to those of mastitis.

Abscesses don't go away on their own, and in fact tend to need hospital treatment. They can only be diagnosed by ultrasound, so a referral to a breast clinic is what usually happens.

You will be advised to carry on breastfeeding even if you have an abscess, and it's important that you do, if at all possible. You will need to make sure you've got good support around you.

As with blocked ducts, there are many other causes of breast lumps, of course, so please do get checked out if you ever find any.

General guidance for avoiding breast problems

For most of the problems above, there is some general guidance to help prevent them.

- **Position and latch.** I know, I know I keep banging on about this through the book, but it's because it's really key to so much! If the baby isn't positioned or latched at the breast in a way that means they can effectively feed, the breast won't get drained and problems can arise.

- **Frequent feeds**. If there is a longer gap than usual between feeds, or a missed feed, you are at higher risk of engorgement, blocked ducts and mastitis. It's important to feed on demand, and if your baby naturally starts to go longer between feeds at any point, you may need to hand express just enough so that your breasts feel comfortable.

- **Avoid tummy sleeping**. Unfortunately for tummy sleepers, this can put pressure on refilling breasts and make them unhappy. Best avoided, if possible!

- **Well-fitting bra**. A bra (or clothing) that puts pressure on the breast is another risk factor for blockages and mastitis.

- **Avoid creating oversupply**. Over the last few years, we've seen a huge increase in people with a true oversupply of milk, i.e. having much more milk than their baby needs. This seems to be linked to the increase in use of one-piece silicone pumps or 'let-down catchers', which are attached to one side while feeding on the other. These do draw off more milk than just catching what's leaked, and as such signal to the body that more milk is needed. Having too much milk can cause all manner of problems and really isn't pleasant. I'd avoid use of these, especially in the first six to eight weeks, if at all possible. There's also no need to pump for a freezer stash!

- **Correct pump sizing**. Expressing with a pump that doesn't fit well can cause nipple damage, and stop the breast from draining effectively. If you're pumping for any reason, visit p. 142 for tips on flange sizing and how to make sure pumping goes well.

- **Avoid using nipple shields, if possible**. Nipple shields, especially if not applied or sized correctly, have the potential to stop milk from draining well. If you're using a shield, it's hugely important to have skilled support to make sure things are going well. See p. 79 for more on this.

- **Look after yourself**. High stress, and being 'run down', appear to have a link with higher rates of mastitis. It can be incredibly difficult to get enough time for self-care when you have a baby, but it's important to prioritise it, if you can. Try to eat well, and rest when you can. Make sure to ask for support from those around you as well.

- **Mental health support**. Parents who have mental health struggles when they've had a baby have higher rates of mastitis. It might be that you already struggled with your mental health before you had the baby, or it may be that it's something that's happened since they arrived. Either way, it does put you at higher risk, so it's really important to make sure you seek help with your mental health.

- **Getting help sooner rather than later**. This goes for anything and everything after having the baby. If you have any worries, questions, doubts, pains . . . get help. Don't let things get worse.

Could it be thrush?

A breastfeeding problem that gets suggested often in the early weeks is thrush.

Thrush is a fungal infection that can affect both your baby's mouth, and your breasts. However, we have a real problem with thrush being diagnosed and treated, but problems not resolving. And that's because it actually wasn't thrush!

Let me explain a bit more.

Parents often report their baby has been given thrush treatment because they've got a white tongue, but that the treatment isn't working. That's because what's actually caused this is milk. In a baby's mouth, thrush looks like white patches, a bit like cottage cheese, and these will not be just on the tongue. It will quickly spread to all over the mouth, including gums, lips and inside the cheeks.

When a baby doesn't have a deep latch, milk doesn't get wiped off the tongue in the same way during the feed and can build up into quite a thick residue. This can then look a lot like thrush might, but it isn't the same at all. If you're offered thrush treatment for whiteness on the tongue that isn't anywhere else in the mouth, ask for a swab to confirm it is actually a fungal infection.

Something else that's inside a baby's mouth that gets mistaken for thrush is some little white blisters that can appear on the roof of the mouth, or along the gums, called Epstein pearls. These are very common in new babies (up to 85 per cent). These are actually benign cysts caused by build-up of keratin, similar to the milk rash that some babies get. The way you can tell Epstein pearls apart from thrush is that they are defined white spots rather than patches, and if they're on the roof of the mouth, they will be along the middle.

For parents, we may be given thrush treatment for nipple and breast pain, especially if our baby has a white tongue, but, as above, this is actually a latch issue a lot of the time. There can be quite mixed messages about what a decent latch is, and so, unfortunately, we may be told the latch looks great or even perfect, leading us to think the pain must be from something else. So we seek out help and thrush gets misdiagnosed. Again, please do ask for a swab to confirm. I hate that there are so many parents getting diagnosed with the wrong thing, as it really delays us finding the real problem and solving it.

> 'My baby had a thick white coating on his tongue and I had nipple pain that I couldn't get rid of, so I was told it was thrush. I tried loads of different creams for me and for my baby and nothing worked, but I just kept getting told that thrush is really difficult to get rid of and prescribed something else. The health visitor came after a few weeks and told me I wasn't holding him right, so I went online and figured out how to get a better latch and everything got much better. I'm convinced it never was thrush, and I'm upset that I gave my baby loads of drops that he didn't ever need' – Lara, mum of baby Isaac.

That said, some people really do have thrush, though, and here are the facts you need to be able to identify it. Firstly, thrush pain will always come on after a period of pain-free feeding. If your feeds have been consistently uncomfortable since your baby was born, it's very unlikely to be thrush. Secondly, thrush pain happens *after* a feed, every feed, in both breasts. It's like hot needles shooting deep into the breast. Vasospasms (see p. 76) can also feel like this, though, so try to seek out well-trained breast-feeding support to help you understand what the issue might be for you.

To treat diagnosed thrush, you will have a cream for your nipples, and your baby will have oral drops or gel. You will both need to be treated regardless of which one of you has it.

> 'We'd been feeding happily for a couple of months and then I started to feel like there were razor blades in my nipples, I couldn't figure out what was going on. Then I noticed Zak's mouth had a load of white creamy stuff inside his cheeks. We got treatment and it cleared pretty quickly.' – Alice, mum of Zak.

Conclusion

Breast problems can be tricky, but what makes it harder is if you can't figure out what's going on, or if you're given the wrong information. I understand how hugely frustrating it can be to feel like you're getting given wrong answers, and I really wish I could change it! Hopefully this book will give you some ideas of what may or may not be happening for you and how best to manage it.

Remember that an IBCLC is going to be really well placed to help you with your own situation too. They're boob detectives!

Christina's story

A few people mentioned that breastfeeding could be difficult, and while I nodded my head in understanding, I sort of thought, 'Yeah, okay. It is the natural way, though, and the human race has survived this far . . .' I think the truest thing I heard was that breastfeeding is natural like walking, not like breathing. I was beyond lucky to be surrounded by a wonderful group of seven other new mums, whom I met through NCT, and we all faced some different obstacles in our feeding journey, as there was blood, sweat and – in every case – tears in those initial weeks. Spoiler alert: seven months in, we are all still breastfeeding our babies. So, the second truth I learned was that breastfeeding, 'learning to walk', is for sure difficult, but that women are *strong*. Possibly the only thing stronger than a woman, these last months have taught me, is the effect of a group of women banding together in support of one another. WhatsApp conversations at 2am, glasses (bottles) of wine and endless empathy, and the capacity to joke about the shittiest of days. More powerful than any nipple cream I tried.

Hamish and I learned to feed and it was all worth it, not that our journey was particularly difficult. We had misdiagnosed thrush and reflux, but after ten weeks we were doing just fine un-medicated and I learned to trust my intuition on these things.

Then when Hamish was four months old, I left him at bedtime for the first time to go riding with a friend. I was thrown off my horse and broke my neck as I hit the ground. The following hours were spent being endlessly x-rayed and scanned. I was told I could end up paralysed and unable to look after my baby. I was strapped to a hospital bed, where I wailed for my baby solidly for eight hours. Labour had nothing on that night. My husband was not allowed in due to Covid, but in the end they bent the rules in the hope he could calm me down (he couldn't). A midwife was brought in to pump me every couple of hours while we waited for results. I remember crying as the milk she pumped pooled around my back (as I was strapped down, the milk couldn't be collected, and would never feed my baby, who it was meant for). Knowing that was utterly heartbreaking. I felt like the worst mum ever and bargained – with who, I don't know – that if I could hold and feed my son one more time, I wouldn't ask for anything else, ever.

Finally, at 3am, I was home with my baby. CT scans showed I wasn't paralysed, and I had no brain damage, so I was strapped into a hard neck brace to allow my multiple fractures to heal. I couldn't move my neck at all, and could only look straight ahead. I felt so guilty for leaving my baby, and for getting into the accident in the first place, that people's helpful suggestions to offer my son formula – given my injuries and difficulty moving – were inconceivable to me. I couldn't pick him up or cuddle him, so producing milk felt like the one thing my body was still capable of. Hamish fed on demand, so his dad or granny (both absolute saints) would sit me up and latch him on and off every couple of hours, day and night.

On the fourth day, at 4am, I texted Lucy in some despair, as I was in so much pain from being propped up to feed, and yet breastfeeding meant more to me than ever. I couldn't stop, I just couldn't. Even over video call, Lucy helped us come up with positions for me to feed Hamish in lying down, and told me I could get through it and feed my baby for a long time to come.

[And she did! Three months later, Christina had her neck brace removed, and she and Hamish continued to breastfeed until he was seventeen months old. Christina made a full recovery.]

8
Expressing

I expect loads of you will want or need this chapter! Expressing has become a big part of breastfeeding for a lot of parents during their journey. We've touched on expressing already, but let's get right back to basics here – what is it?

Expressing is when you take some milk from the breast by hand, or breast pump. This might be to feed the baby, to store, to help increase supply, or for lots of other reasons.

Although a lot of people express, please don't feel it's something you have to do if you don't want to. Certainly, during pregnancy you may have assumed you'll combine expressing with breast-feeding, but in reality is that what you'll want or need? Maybe, maybe not!

We may think it's a simple activity, but in reality expressing can take time and practice and there are a few things to take into consideration. But that's why this chapter is here! To help you think it through and get the most out of expressing (Badaboom-tish!), if it's something you choose to do.

Hand expressing

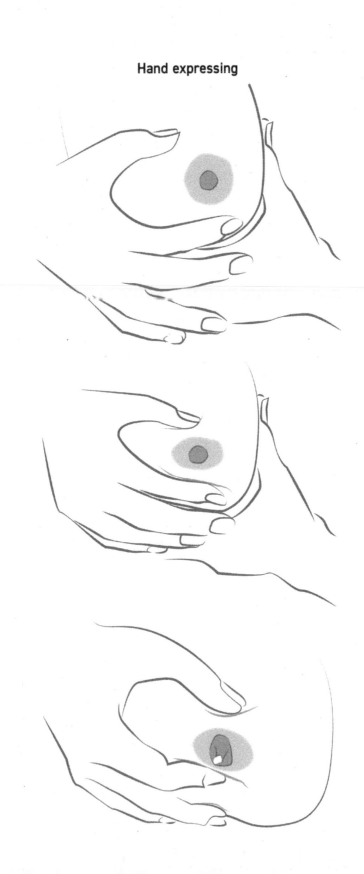

Hand expressing

Hand expressing is something I would strongly recommend you learn. It's a way of removing milk from the breast – you guessed it – by hand! No tools required.

It's a really handy thing to know how to do, not only because it can be an effective way of removing milk, but also because you can do it anywhere with minimal to no planning/prep required. You can also target specific areas more easily by hand, so if you had a blocked duct, for example, you'd be able to work more directly on that area.

So how do you do it? Well, the most important thing is to remember that it should be a relaxing and comfortable experience. Try not to think of it as a 'procedure', but more as just a part of something natural that you do. While there is a technique you can use, it will vary slightly for everyone, and whatever you find works best for you is fine!

Try making a C shape with your thumb and first two fingers. Feel back from your nipple until you feel a change; a firmer, lumpy texture. This is the spot you'll be compressing.

Using the C shape you've created, compress for a couple of seconds in a firm but comfortable way and then release for a couple of seconds. Repeat. Build up this slow, steady rhythm without dragging the skin or causing discomfort. It can take a bit of time for the colostrum to come, or you may need to move your C shape back or forward ever so slightly until you 'hit the spot'.

Some people find a gentle roll forward with your fingers can be useful. Others may find pushing back a little toward the chest wall before compressing helpful.

There are ducts all the way around the breast so once you've finished the first spot you can move your C shape around to a different place.

Antenatal hand expressing

In the last few weeks of pregnancy (36 weeks onward, usually, but speak to your midwife), some parents choose to start hand expressing. This is useful so as to get some colostrum stored in the freezer, in case for some reason the baby needs extra milk, or you aren't able to feed (as we covered on p. 17).

I'm a big fan of this, because not only does it give you a bit of a 'safety net' of extra milk, should you need it, but, really importantly, it helps you learn how to hand express before your baby arrives.

Imagine the baby has arrived but won't latch and you've been advised to express some colostrum: you'd be able to go bosh! Got some! Rather than, erm, how do I do that? And then feel pressured and stressed. Plus, if you do have a baby that is a bit reluctant to feed in those first few days, you'll be able to provide the colostrum they need, and also stimulate your breasts and therefore supply. So, yep, I'm fully on board if you want to have a go at this.

It is important to remember that colostrum is produced in very small quantities, though, so we're not looking for ounces and ounces of milk to be expressed. For most people it will take a bit of time and practice to get anything, then perhaps a glistening on the nipple at most, then a drop or two, then perhaps a millilitre or so as time goes on. That's completely normal! So when we talk about storing some colostrum antenatally, we're talking about perhaps a few little syringes full. And if you don't get that, or any, please don't worry. It is *not* an indicator of future milk supply at all.

Colostrum starts to be made midway through pregnancy, and doesn't change to the next stage of milk production until the placenta is born, so rest assured there's no worries about it being somehow used up or running out before the baby gets here. Most people express directly into a syringe, or into a clean container and then suck it up with the syringe to store. You can usually get syringes with caps/lids from your midwife or GP surgery, and you can also buy kits online.

Remember to label them individually with your name and date of birth (so that they can be identified as yours if they're taken to hospital) and put them into a clean bag or tub before freezing (we don't want them rolling around in the bottom of the freezer with stray frozen peas!). You don't necessarily need to take your syringes with you to the hospital, especially if you know someone will be able to bring them to you if they are needed. If you do decide to take your supply in, make sure you transport it with ice packs and let your maternity team know immediately on arrival that you need it put in the freezer. You could even check with your maternity department during your pregnancy that they have a freezer available for this, just in case.

Why hand expressing and not a pump at this stage? Because colostrum is thick, sticky, and comes in very small amounts. A pump just isn't as effective as hand expressing for colostrum.

{*If you choose to express during pregnancy, please check with your health provider, and please stop if you have any discomfort or tummy aches*}

'I really think doing this in those last few weeks of pregnancy was what made breastfeeding work for us. I felt like I understood how my breasts worked so much better, and even though I didn't need to use the bits of colostrum I'd frozen, it was still really nice to know it was there' – Jaime, parent to Daniel.

Pumping

Pumping is another way of expressing milk. This is when you use what's basically a special gadget to remove the milk rather than just your hands. There are lots of different pumps you can get hold of, from manual (which you squeeze by hand), electric (which does the suction for you), single or double (meaning expressing one side or both sides at once), wireless, wearable pumps, and one-piece silicone 'let down catchers', which you can see more about below.

How do I know which pump to get?

There are tons of different brands on the market, and it can seem a bit overwhelming to say the least! So it can be useful to think about what you want a pump for. Is it for occasional use, or will you be pumping daily? Is it to increase milk supply? Is it for pumping at work? Will you have access to electricity? It can be worth waiting until your baby has arrived before you get a pump, so that you know what you need it for.

Remember, too, that more expensive does not necessarily equal better with pumps.

If it's just for occasional use, you can choose whichever is within your budget and you like the look of, but it's really important that the pump is the right fit for you. See more about flange sizing below. It's also helpful to choose one that's a 'closed system', so it can be reused in the future. Closed systems have a barrier between the pump mechanism and milk collection parts, and so there is less chance of contamination, for example from mould.

If you're using a pump to increase milk supply, a 'hospital grade' electric pump is the most effective, but they're expensive, so it's worth looking into hiring rather than buying. Whatever you get, a double pump is important when increasing supply. And, again, flange sizing is vital.

Wireless pumps that you wear in your bra have become very popular over the last few years. They are extremely convenient in that you're able to carry on and do other things at the same time, or pump on the go, and people really like that. But, I'm not the biggest fan, if I'm honest. It seems very difficult to get the correct flange sizing with wireless pumps, perhaps because they're a fairly new product. Maybe this will change. I hope so. And flange sizing is so important – again, see below!

For some people, wearable pumps work really well; however, lots of parents tell me they don't get as much as with other pumps. They're definitely not good for parents who are trying to increase supply. They also have a tendency to leak, and that stuff is PRECIOUS. 'No use crying over spilled milk'? The heck there is!

But my main worry is that wearable pumps buy into the narrative of the 'supermum', that we can constantly multitask and run around doing all the things for everyone all the time.

Nah, I want to sit my bum down and read a book and eat some chocolate while I pump, thanks! I'm doing important work, and my time and effort should be valued.

If you have a friend or family member that has a pump (closed system) that you can try before you buy, do that! But remember to clean and sterilise before use and before you give it back. And keep in mind that you may have to buy/try several different pumps before you find the right one for you.

How to get the most out of pumping

It's not just about the pump!

Pumping needs to be as relaxing and comfortable as possible. As important as breast stimulation is, it's also vital that your hormones can flow to let the milk out. This won't happen (as easily) if you're feeling tense, stressed or upset. Don't just think about the mechanics of getting the milk out, think about your mental and emotional state too. Now isn't the time to be worrying about whether grandad likes his birthday socks! You want to do things that make you feel happier, 'loved up' and maybe even want to laugh. For me, a cup of tea, some chocolate, and an episode of *Friends* on the box would be ideal!

Other things that can encourage that hormone and milk flow can be useful, such as watching videos of your little one feeding, or sniffing some of their clothes! Pumping on one side while feeding on the other is a great way of getting milk flowing if you have the option too.

Breast massage before pumping is yet another great way of getting hormones flowing and encouraging milk ejection. Gentle, comfortable massage helps you to relax, and it also mimics how your little one may paw at or bob on and off the breast at first, making it feel a lot more like breastfeeding. Continuing to use a 'hands on' technique while pumping has been found to really increase the amount expressed. Massage, and gentle compression, may be useful to target areas that still feel firmer with milk, but also to elicit other 'let downs'.

Covering the bottle with something so that you can't see what you're expressing is a great hack, I find. It stops you focusing on what's come out and stressing about amounts.

Pumps don't last for ever! In fact, it's recommended that you replace the valves in the pump fairly often. Check your own pump instructions to see what the manufacturer recommends. It depends how often you're using it, of course, but every few months is usual if it's being used often. But if the amounts you're expressing start to decrease, have a think whether pump parts may need replacing.

How long do I pump for?

This varies from person to person. Some people can easily access lots of milk in the first five minutes, whereas others haven't even had their 'let down' by that point.

Once your 'let down' has happened, whenever that may be, around 10 to 20 minutes of pumping after that is average, but for some people it will take longer. The main thing is to have a look and see what's happening with flow – if the flow has subsided, you won't get much milk after that, unless you can elicit another 'let down', so you may wish to stop or take a break and do some breast massage or hand expressing to get some last valuable drops.

How often should I pump?

That depends on the reason you're pumping! If you're aiming to increase your supply, then six to eight times in 24 hours is advisable, including once at night. If you're pumping to store some milk before your return to work, for example, then once may be fine, depending on when you go back. If you're exclusively pumping for all feeds, however, it's most likely you'll need to pump ten to twelve times for each 24-hour period.

Flange sizing

The flange of a pump is the part that actually makes contact with the breast, and that the nipple goes into. These can be different shapes and sizes, and it's really important that the right size is used. This is for comfort, but also for maximising the amount of milk and the effectiveness and efficiency.

Pump companies usually include only one or two sizes, and they tend to be large ones, presumably to make sure everyone fits in. Unfortunately, we often assume we should just use the flanges provided because they must be correct, but actually they may not be effective or comfortable at all, and are often far too big.

Traditionally, we were told to make sure the nipple fitted in the flange with a few millimetres space all the way around, but now we're starting to recognise that actually a snugger fit is usually more effective. It would seem the key is to get the smallest size you can that is comfortable (genuinely comfortable, not just 'I can put up with this' level of comfort) and that maximises the amount of milk and potentially sprays that are coming. Some pump companies have different size flanges that you can order, but, if not, or they don't fit or work for you, you can also order flange inserts to get the right fit. Just don't underestimate how important flange sizing is for pumping!

> 'I was such a rubbish pumper, I'd just get a dribble. I really needed to get some milk in the freezer for an early return back to work, so I spoke with an IBCLC, who helped me check my pump fit. Game changer! So much more enjoyable to pump, and I actually started getting sprays!' – Kelly, mum to Ffion.

Let-down catchers

A 'let-down catcher' is a type of one-piece pump where you feed on one side and suction the pump onto the other breast while you do so. The idea is that it catches what you leak from the other side while you feed. Potentially a very nifty, easy, effective and low-cost gadget. However, they do come with drawbacks, that I touched on on p. 123.

Let-down catchers suction onto the breast, first of all, so they do actually remove more milk than you would leak during a feed. And removing milk leads to making more milk, so, if you were to use one of these often, you could potentially end up with too much milk supply, which really isn't as good as it sounds. This is particularly likely to be a problem if you use them in the first six weeks, when milk supply is only really getting established. My other concern is that I've seen people compromise their position and latch on the feeding side to make sure the pump is suctioned on, and that in itself can cause real problems. So I'd say: use with caution.

Can I express in the first six weeks?

There's a lot online about not expressing in the first six weeks after a baby is born, and I see a lot of misinformation shared, so I'll try and clear it up here. In that first six weeks or so, your body is working hard to get your milk supply established and regulate itself to what your baby needs. So, ideally, you want to try to avoid expressing, or much expressing, in those early weeks, as you would be signalling to your body to make more milk than you need. While that may sound good, having an oversupply is actually a really horrible problem. Feeding can become difficult, blocked ducts and mastitis are more common, babies struggle more with wind . . . and more. So you want to try and avoid an oversupply, if you can.

Now, that's not to say you can't express at all. Your boobs won't fall off or anything! And certainly, some people do need to express, for reasons such as feeding plans and increasing milk supply. It's that we want to express through necessity rather than choice in those first few weeks, if possible.

'My boobs were no joke. They were constantly full even like an hour after I'd fed. I was permanently leaking and having to change my clothes several times a day. My baby would struggle with how much milk I had, coming off coughing and choking, and he was often really sick after he'd fed. It was like he wanted to feed for comfort but just got too much milk, all the time. He had a gripey tummy and explosive poo, which I'm sure were linked with it too. It was a pretty miserable start. Ironically, I'd pumped loads in the beginning because I was so worried I wouldn't have enough milk.' – Tal, mum to Farah.

That said, I'm a big believer in simply doing what you need to do to get through. We have a lot of people stopping breastfeeding before they'd plan in those early days because it can be tough and support is minimal. So, if you need to express on occasion for someone else to feed, and it stops you from stopping breast-feeding before you wanted, go for it! Just keep it to a minimum, and try to find other ways of getting help and support if you can too.

When is the best time to express?

A lot of parents find morning is the most productive time to express. It seems that there's more 'available' milk kicking around and it's more easily accessible. But the best time is really when you have the time, energy, and the brain space to do it! Remember how important that hormone flow and relaxation is, so try to pick a time when you can really make it work.

Should you express before, after or at the same time as a feed? Well, I guess it depends on why you're expressing. If it's to boost supply, then after a feed is useful. If it's to get some milk for a feed or to build a stash, then at the same time or after. If you're doing it for a freezer stash, for example, try to do it around the same time daily, so that your body gets used to what you're asking of it.

What's a normal amount to express?

I can guarantee it's not as much as you expect! We see images from breast pump companies with big bottles full of milk, and in reality it's not that way for most people. Around 30–90ml (1–3 oz) is fairly normal, depending on your situation and storage capacity. Remember that what you can pump is *not* an indication of your supply! And you may also find that one breast will give you more milk than the other.

What's storage capacity?

The amount of milk that can be stored in the breast varies from person to person, and even from breast to breast! Some people can store a huge amount, others very little. And, nope, the size of your breasts has absolutely nothing to do with your storage capacity.

If you have small storage capacity, does that mean you can't make enough milk? Not at all. It just means your baby may want to feed more frequently.

Think of it this way: you and a couple of friends decided to focus on drinking two litres of water a day. You have a small cup. Your first friend has a large cup. Your second friend has a massive mug. You can all drink two litres, but you'd have to refill way more often than your mates.

How do I know what my storage capacity is? Well, you don't, really, and, actually, it doesn't usually matter. But it can be helpful to know variation exists as part of normal physiology, and is one of the reasons that some babies feed more frequently than others, and why some people get more off than others when expressing.

Do I need a freezer stash?

This is huge on social media, with people sharing pics of their massive freezer stashes in what sometimes seems almost a competitive way! But do you really need one? No, almost certainly not. There are very few reasons where you would need to store a lot. The saying goes 'feed the baby, not the freezer'.

I'm not suggesting you don't store milk, of course you can – it's one of the many beauties of breastmilk, that it can freeze, which is hugely convenient – but please don't feel you have to be busting your guts trying to express for a huge stash.

> 'I felt so much pressure to get loads of milk in my freezer. I didn't even need it, it was just something that I felt you had to do. I hated pumping, it took me away from time with my baby, and it felt really unnatural to me to be strapped up to the machine.

> 'I broke down one day saying that I was really finding it too hard to fit everything in and I was feeling like a terrible mum. I decided I'd slow it down and stop expressing and it felt amazing. I felt so free after that.'

How much milk will they need?

If you're planning on giving some expressed milk to your breast-fed baby, as I've said above, ideally try to avoid doing so, if possible, until they're around six weeks or so. But remember that this is *your* baby and *your* feeding journey.

From around one month to six months old, your baby takes on average the same amount of milk each day. Yep! Seems crazy, doesn't it, given that they're growing so fast, but rather than increasing in volume, breastmilk adapts to their needs in composition.

The average milk intake in 24 hours is around 750ml (25 ounces). So if you calculate how many times your baby feeds, roughly, over 24 hours, you should be able to work out how much to offer as a feed. For example, if your baby feeds ten times, it may be 75ml (2.5 ounces) for a feed. There are a few other things to take into consideration, though!

We usually recommend offering 120ml (4 ounces) as a maximum for a breastfed baby. The reason for this is that it's very unlikely they would take this amount directly from the breast, and so, if they have too much, it could stretch their tummy and make them uncomfortable, and also it could lead to them being unsatisfied with smaller amounts when they're back at the breast. After all, bottle feeding is very different to breastfeeding (see more below).

If they've taken the expected amount of milk and are still unsettled, it may be that they're seeking the comfort and soothing of the breastfeed. You can either pop them back on the boob to settle, or whoever else is feeding them can perhaps offer a clean finger to suck, or you can rock or bounce them to soothe.

Bottle feeding a breastfed baby

Remember that feeding is not just about milk but also about relaxation, connection and comfort, and often sleep too! It's a good idea to offer a bottle feed with what's known as a 'paced' technique. Partly to ensure the feed is relaxed, but also because the actual act of moving milk is different with a bottle, and often a lot faster. If they feed too fast, not only will they not recognise that they've finished feeding and will keep showing feeding cues, but they could also end up windy and bloated.

Comfortable, paced feeding position

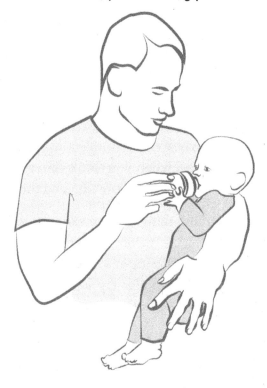

Standard position, but may cause fast or over-feeding

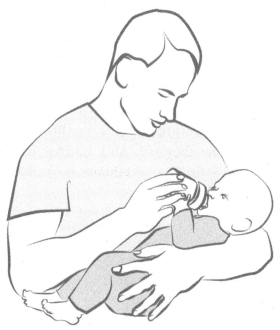

Why is my baby refusing a bottle?

Some babies really aren't a fan of having a bottle. Ultimately, it's not something they need to know how to do biologically, so their instincts may well be to reject it in favour of the breast. It makes sense when you think about it, but it can be difficult when you want to use one and they won't!

The most important thing is to make sure feeding is a relaxing experience, so never ever force it. Time and patience are key. Try offering at a time that they're not too hungry or tired. You can also try warming the teat so it feels more similar to the breast temperature.

Some babies won't ever take a bottle, but from around four months old, they can start having milk from a cup. In the meantime, you may need to find other ways around your challenges, such as going out straight after a feed, or having them brought to you for a feed while you're at work.

Is there a bottle that's best for a breastfed baby?

Nope. You'll see it written on the packaging of bottles, for sure, but that's just advertising. There is *no* brand of bottle that's best, no matter what they say. All I'd advise is that you find one that's affordable for you, and that feels comfortable to hold for a long time!

Exclusive expressing

One option for feeding your baby is to exclusively express. That means not putting them to the breast at all, and giving your expressed breastmilk via a bottle. There are a few reasons why parents may do this, and one is through choice – it may just fit best with that particular family and that's the way they prefer to feed. Another is if direct feeding hasn't worked out for them, for example if the baby wasn't ever able to latch. There are also some babies that are in NICU for a long time – for example, very premature babies – and because they're apart a lot, mum pumps to leave milk. There are pros and cons to exclusive expressing. But, as with everything, the cons are minimised with the right support and information.

How long can expressed milk be stored?

Freshly expressed milk can be kept at room temperature for up to six hours. It can be kept in the main part of the fridge (not in the door), meanwhile, for up to six to eight days, as long as your fridge is 4°C (39°F) or less. If you don't know, or it's warmer than this, use within three days. Give it a sniff before you use it, as you'll know if it's gone off – it's milk!

It can be kept in the freezer compartment of a fridge for two weeks, though, or in a deep freeze for up to six months (–18°C / 0°F or lower).

Top tip: freeze in amounts of 60–90ml (2–3 ounces) maximum to avoid waste.

Milk that has been defrosted should be used within 24 hours (to defrost milk, the ideal way is to slowly do it in the fridge over several hours, but you can also sit the bottle or bag in some hot water if you need it more quickly). If your freezer power goes out, don't open the freezer door. As long as there are still ice crystals in the milk once the power returns, it can be safely frozen again and used. If it's fully defrosted, sadly it should be used or discarded.

Once milk has been offered to the baby, it should be used within an hour, and after that the unused portion should be discarded or put into their bath! Yep, unused or out of date milk is lovely and moisturising in the bath.

Milk donation

Something else you may wish to express for is to donate your milk. Humans have shared milk with each other for most likely thousands of years. While some parents do still feed each other's babies directly, or express to share with friends and family, the most common form of milk donation is to a milk bank.

Milk banks are facilities that screen, store and distribute human milk to premature or unwell babies, usually in NICU units. We know only too well that human milk makes the most incredible difference to the lives and health of these babies, and that it's not possible without their generous donors.

The process usually involves you making contact with your local donation centre. Sadly some places don't have one locally, but often those further afield are happy to transport the milk. They usually want to screen you first, including blood tests and questionnaires to make sure not only that you're suitable, but also that, mentally speaking, it's going to be appropriate. While we know donor milk is important, we also know that *you* are important, and donating is a generous gift that needs to be manageable and not cause you distress.

Once screened, you'll usually be given the equipment needed, and instructions about how and where to store the milk. Once you've reached a certain amount, the milk can be collected and taken for pasteurising.

> 'James was around four months old when I felt like we were finally in our rhythm with feeding. I saw on Instagram a post about donating milk and it felt like the right thing to do. It wasn't always easy at times, and there were days when I really didn't have the energy, but when I handed over that first donation it felt wonderful to know I was helping poorly babies.' – Pippa and baby James.

Conclusion

Hopefully that's helped you clear up some of the ins and outs of expressing: it's not quite as straightforward as it seems, huh? But it can be such a valuable tool when used in the right way, and I know a lot of parents would say they couldn't have breastfed, or breastfed for as long, without expressing. I also know many that would say it was just too much of a faff and they quickly knocked it on the head.

Either way, you'll find the right path for you, but, as with all of this, I hope you're recognising by now that the right support makes a huge difference.

Gemma's story

After a long battle to conceive, I had my heart set on exclusively breastfeeding; it just meant so much to me. Unfortunately, with PCOS and IGT, exclusively breastfeeding wasn't going to happen and it took me a long time to come to terms with that. I felt inadequate, like I wasn't fulfilling my role as a mother, and at first I thought I was going to have to stop as I didn't realise I could combination feed long term. It just wasn't talked about as an option! I was met with dismissive comments from well-meaning friends and family who just didn't understand how important it was to me, but, thankfully, I found a support network who really drove me forward and educated me. I wanted to protect breastfeeding as much as possible, so we ensured we paced our bottle feeds and used an at-the-breast supplementary nursing system (SNS) in the early months, which was a little faffy but great to get formula into my baby as well as stimulating my supply. For me, the SNS wasn't a long-term solution, but once I was happy that breastfeeding was well established, I stopped using it. I continued to breastfeed my daughter until she was almost three-and-a-half years old.

With my second baby, supply was better but still not sufficient, and eventually it got to the point where I knew I had to supplement. I'd educated myself a lot since my first baby, so I knew of the many benefits breastmilk had to offer. This time, instead of introducing formula straight away, I asked some of my friends if they were willing to donate some of their breastmilk to help us along the way. I was overwhelmed with the response and it went a long way to help heal the wounds of not having a full supply. And here we are, at eighteen months, still going strong. I've learned there's so much more to breastfeeding than just the milk, and for us it became a lot more about comfort and connecting with each other.

9
Reflux

During these early months, babies can go through a lot, and it can be hard to unpick what's normal and what's a problem. Reflux is a term that you'll most likely hear bandied about, and you may well be wondering if that's what's going on with your baby, so I thought it would be helpful to discuss it here, and also discuss what may *look* like reflux, but is actually something else, or may even be normal.

What is reflux?

Reflux is a term used to describe babies who regurgitate their tummy contents and spit up (i.e. are sick). And it's actually pretty common, and almost always normal.

At two months old, almost 87 per cent of babies spit up every day. At four months, this is down to just under 70 per cent. By six months it's under half.

Some babies spit up a little bit after feeds, and this is known as posseting. Some do occasional bigger vomits too. Both can be normal.

Reflux doesn't usually cause babies pain or distress. Perhaps momentary unpleasantness, but that's usually all. Reflux happens, in essence, because babies are on a fully liquid diet, feed a *lot*, and don't have very much in the way of strength or maturity to their tummy muscles or valves to hold it in. Spitting up also helps protect them from over feeding – if they've taken too much milk, they just let a bit out! (NB: you know when you're pregnant and people tell you to buy lots of muslin cloths? Yeah, *this* is why!)

What's 'silent reflux'?

'Silent reflux' is when they regurgitate their tummy contents, but swallow it back down again (yuck – sorry!). It's called 'silent' because it's happening but there isn't any visible evidence of it in the way of spit up. They might pull a bit of a funny face when it happens, or be a bit miffed for a bit, but, overall, it shouldn't bother them much. Again, for the most part, silent reflux is part and parcel of being a baby. And babies can have reflux *and* silent reflux at the same time.

Is it a problem?

It can certainly be messy, I won't lie. Some babies can be pretty pukey. For most families this is the biggest problem with reflux: the mess and the laundry. But as long as your baby is growing well, filling nappies as expected, and you're not having any feeding problems, reflux is something that will resolve itself as they get older and bigger. If there is any green staining or blood in their sick, however, seek urgent help.

What can I do to help?

Well, firstly, the most important thing is knowing that you're not doing anything wrong and that, overwhelmingly, reflux is normal and not in the least bit sinister. The vast majority of babies' symptoms improve as the weeks and months go by.

In the meantime, things that can help are lots of skin-to-skin cuddles. Skin to skin releases feel-good hormones, and is soothing and comforting. Not just for the baby, but for you as well!

Frequent feeds also help. Some babies can be better feeding 'little and often', which can be easier for digestion. Or simply the act of feeding may be helpful and comforting, or support them with sleep.

Carrying them, ideally using a sling or carrier, so that they're held close and upright (facing inwards to you), is worth trying too. Babies that are carried in slings are known to cry less, grow faster, and parents report better mental health for themselves.

'Tummy time', meanwhile, where babies spend short bursts of time lying on their front while supervised, helps strengthen core muscles, which in turn can support reduction of reflux. And baby massage has been found to help too!

But my main suggestion, as with pretty much all baby-related challenges, would be to look at the support network around you and think holistically. Who can help with cooking, cleaning, shopping? Who can hold the baby while you nap? Who would be a helpful person if you're in need of an emotional outpouring to a listening ear? This, truly, is what will make the biggest difference. Reach out to those around you, as it's too much to deal with alone.

Gastro-oesophageal reflux disease

For some babies, however, their reflux can be a significant problem – gastro-oesophageal reflux disease or GORD – though this is rarer than perhaps it would seem, with some sources suggesting only 1 in 300 babies. For the babies in question, the vomiting can be excessive, in both frequency and amount, and can often be projectile. Their condition can have an impact on their weight gain and growth, their nappies, and these babies can become extremely distressed, unsettled and unhappy, often seeming like they're in a lot of pain a lot of the time. Any baby diagnosed with this condition should receive specialist input.

A baby with GORD will need a lot of care; frequent feeds and babywearing are your friends. Over and above a specialised feeding assessment and plan, some families may be offered a trial of medications. The medical professionals should discuss with you, in full, the benefits and risks of these medications, though, so that you can make an informed decision, as it's important to be aware that the evidence for how well these treatments work is mixed. It's also important to know that GORD is actually a symptom, and treatments, if started, should be short term and not detract from discovering the underlying cause. While I'll outline medications briefly below, it's incredibly important that you discuss treatment options fully with your care team.

Reflux medications

There are three main types of medications that get prescribed for reflux: feed thickeners, alginate therapy, and acid suppression.

Feed thickeners are a substance that gets added to milk to thicken it, and, in theory, reduce what gets regurgitated. These are not compatible with breastfeeding and so tend only to be described to bottle-feeding parents.

Alginate therapy comes up more often, and the most common of these is known by the brand name Gaviscon. The medication gets mixed with some milk and given to the baby, and is believed to form a sort of thick cover on top of the stomach contents to hold it down.

It can be very difficult to give to a breastfed baby, however, and can cause constipation, so it's not uncommon for families to move away from this medication quite quickly.

If Gaviscon isn't working, or the side effects are too difficult to manage, the next step would be a **proton pump inhibitor** – also known as an acid suppressant, an example being Omeprazole. If you're prescribed this treatment, it's worth investigating the potential side effects in detail, as some of them can be serious. I don't tell you this to scare you, it's just important for you to know that the benefit of taking the treatment must outweigh the risks.

Does my baby need medication?

Whether to medicate or not is really tricky, I know. In the UK, we have lots of babies on medications for reflux, and it can be very hard to know if that's what should be happening for your baby too.

The UK national guidance for babies with reflux is to have a full feeding assessment (not just a latch check) with a trained specialist. This is because simple changes to how and when a baby is fed can dramatically alter what's happening. Giving parents an understanding of what's normal behaviour and what's not and how to manage it is extremely helpful too.

They can also help you find any underlying cause to what's going on, such as allergy, for example, and explain how to manage this. In actual fact, many parents find that they don't need to start medications once they've worked with a feeding specialist.

My advice is that, if you're offered medication for your baby, it's always worth asking for a referral to the infant feeding team and/ or working with an IBCLC first, if you can.

Is it reflux . . . or something else?

Babies can be hard to work out in the early months, and there are a lot of signs or behaviours that can be attributed to reflux, which, in fact, might be due to something else, or just plain normal! Let's have a look at some of the more common behaviours and their causes.

– Frequent feeding

In the first few months, it is normal for a baby to want to feed very frequently. Sometimes upward of twelve times in 24 hours. Feeds are unlikely to be at regular intervals too, say every three hours. It's more likely that they will be quite random, with more frequent feeds at some points, and bigger gaps at others, and there almost certainly won't be a predictable pattern. So it may well be normal if your baby is feeding a lot, but, if you feel it's excessive, then revisiting position and latch is the first place to start, and also look at whether your baby is doing enough wee and poo, and gaining weight as expected.

Remember also that babies don't just feed for milk; they feed for comfort, for sleep, for warmth, for connection, and so much more. So it's not a surprise that they want to latch a lot in these first few months when the world is so big and new.

In actual fact, did you know that babies aren't aware they're separate from you until around seven months old? Isn't that amazing? And it explains so much about why babies want to be connected to you so much of the time.

When parents ask me about their baby's unsettled behaviour, I always start by asking if going to the breast settles them. If it's a yes, that's a really good sign that it's normal and not a sign of something like reflux. Okay, it may be a sign that feeding needs adjusting, if they're not able to feed effectively for some reason, but it's usually just because being latched feels like home.

– Unsettled behaviour during feeds

On the whole, babies should be mainly relaxed and comfortable during the majority of feeds. Babies that are fractious during a lot of or all feeds may be that way for a lot of different reasons. Most commonly, it's to do with how they're feeding, meaning that they're either struggling to get fast-enough flow of millk, or, conversely, the flow is too quick. This can cause them to come on and off the breast, or cry, or squirm around while feeding. On p. 62 about growth spurts and cluster feeding: these can cause some really unnerving behaviours, like tugging and latching on and off, and can be completely normal. They're usually fairly short lived, though, so keep that in mind if you're trying to figure out what's happening.

Babies who are not getting enough milk often can be quite unsettled during (and after) feeds, though some fall asleep very quickly into the feed. Again, it can help to go back to chapter 4, and read the passages about getting enough milk, for lots more information about how to tell what's going on here.

It's also worth noting that babies with allergies may have particular difficulties feeding, often due to the discomfort or pain in their tummies from indigestion. See chapter 11 for further reading.

– Temporarily increased needs

Babies regularly appear to go through a type of growth spurt, but for their development rather than physical growth; times when their needs become more intense, while they're working on new skills like smiling, or rolling over – these are often referred to as developmental 'leaps', and they can have an impact on their behaviours at the breast, with sleep, and their temperament. When your fairly happy, relaxed baby suddenly wants to feed all the time, cries a lot, fusses at the breast, wakes up more . . . it's pretty disconcerting, and of course can lead us to thinking something is very wrong. But it may well be a temporary thing related to a 'leap', rather than anything untoward.

Around Weeks 3 to 4 seems to be one of the biggest periods of change for new babies. Parents report more awake time, more crying, more feeding, being a bit less 'easy to please'. So, if this happens to you, remember it's incredibly common and doesn't necessarily mean anything is wrong. Though, of course, if you have any concerns about your baby being unwell you should get them checked over. Rashes, temperatures, refusal to feed, reduced nappy output, or excessive vomiting should all be checked out promptly.

'Anabelle was pretty happy being put in her Moses basket until she was about three-and-a-half weeks old, and then suddenly she changed, she was miserable. Cranky, difficult to please, wanting lots of feeds but unhappy at the breast, not napping as much; it was really difficult, especially as my wife had gone back to work and I was looking after her on my own. I started to get worried that something must be wrong and thought about seeing the GP. Then, about a week later, one morning she started giving her first smiles! She was much happier after that and things calmed back down for a bit.'
– Grace, mum of Anabelle.

– Wanting to be held all the time

As we've discussed in earlier chapters, it's extremely common for new babies to wake when they're put down. It's a survival mechanism! They are completely dependent on their caregivers for pretty much every need – feeding, warmth, comfort, safety; so if they feel that they've been put down, their instinct is to wake back up and signal for help to get safe. They don't know they're in a lovely snuggly space bought specially for them, in their comfy home! So they wake for a safe space, and the place they want is usually back on the boob.

It can be really, *really* exhausting and overwhelming in the early months when they're like this, but it's usually normal (or sometimes the sign of a position and latch issue). But it's not something that should be considered a sign of reflux, though it's one that's commonly suggested! It *does* get easier, I promise, but in the meantime try to get friends and family to help with holding them while you get some rest.

165

– Changes in sleep patterns

On the one hand, we're told that new babies sleep an enormous amount, on the other that we'll be absolutely broken with sleep deprivation. What to believe? What's normal?

In reality, the first few days can be pretty challenging, but for some people things settle down a little after that. You may manage a few chunks of a few hours here or there, which can be surprisingly refreshing and restorative! Around Week 3, though, something seems to change: as we've seen, babies seem to wake up to the world a lot more and are more difficult to get settled. Sometimes this is when the 'not being put down without waking' starts.

Unfortunately, this is also often the point when partners are ending their leave and going back to work, and family and friends have stopped visiting and offering help, whereas it's actually now that we need it most!

These next few weeks are the ones that are the really tough ones sleep-wise. I'm being honest with you, not to scare you, but so that you don't worry that something is really wrong, and because having realistic expectations can help us relax and even cope a bit better, I find. Weeks 3 to 8, in my experience, are usually the ones where people struggle with sleep that bit more. Mainly, I think, because we're expecting things to get easier, and they don't. At least not yet – but they will!

The good news is that around Weeks 10 to 12 is when most parents report the 'best' sleep. Babies start to develop their circadian rhythm, that natural day/night body clock. Often they cluster feed like crazy in the evenings, but, once they settle, they tend to have the longest stretch of sleep, then feed and settle for another long stretch, but shorter than the first (by long, I'm talking three or four hours, by the way). This goes on until about the 4 or 5am mark, which you can read more about below!

– 4am grunting

I expect a lot of you have or will experience this: grunty, groaning, straining, wriggly babies! For some babies, it can happen around the clock, but for most babies it's worse at night, particularly from around 4am onward (if it is around the clock, do get some feeding support, as there may be something going on that can be improved).

It looks so so uncomfortable and distressing, doesn't it? But it often seems even worse for us than for them! It's near on impossible to sleep next to a baby doing this, partly because you spend every other minute wondering if they need feeding or winding, and partly because they're so *loud*!

It's significantly safer for babies to sleep on their backs, so please *please* keep doing this. But for digestion it may not be very helpful, unfortunately, and so, by the early hours of the morning, they're often struggling with wind and poo. Think about it: if you're windy, or have a bit of tummy ache, the last thing you do is lie on your back stretched out, right? But we have to put them on their backs for sleep, so it's something we have to learn to manage for a while. However, it can be extremely unsettling for everyone, because it seems like they're so distressed, and it's *very* disruptive to sleep. The good news is that this too is not a reflux symptom, plus it doesn't last too long and seems to pass around Week 12-ish.

In the meantime, the easiest way to cope with it is to do lots of cuddling! Skin to skin is great, and get some feeding support, as adjustments to how they're feeding can often make a difference as well.

I find that if you have some support that lives with you, it's often easiest to 'tag team' it; i.e. take an hour or two each holding the baby on your chest. We're often reluctant to do this, because it feels like we're giving in and accepting lack of sleep, but, frankly, that's happening anyway, and this way there is less worry and fewer battles. We also know that cuddling babies is really good for their development, physically, mentally and emotionally, so it's a win for everyone.

Oh, and again, I promise you're not 'spoiling them' or 'making a rod for your back' etc etc: babies learn to sleep independently when they're ready.

– Straining (infant dyschezia)

If you see your baby straining, it may not be reflux – they may be trying to pass a poo. In the first few days and weeks, passing poo is often a little easier and it may get passed without drama. As time goes on, though, it seems that babies start to try to coordinate their pooing a bit more, and coordinate the action of their bowels with the pelvic floor muscles. This is a tricky business, and can lead to lots of grunting and straining and going red in the face, sometimes even crying out. It can seem quite uncomfortable! The best way to support them with this, as ever, is with cuddles, and feeding helps too, if they're happy to.

– Back arching

Whenever someone mentions that the baby is arching their back, one of the first things people suggest is reflux. Now, absolutely, if a baby is in discomfort or pain, one of the signs can be that they stiffen and arch their back. However, this may not be reflux pain, and it can also be a sign of many other things too. And if the arching is happening when they're put down, usually it's a sign they need to be held or fed, not of reflux.

– Wind

Wind is common in new babies but isn't linked with reflux. Sometimes gas can cause an occasional bit of vomiting, but on the whole they are two separate things. For more on wind, see p. 174.

> *'Absolutely everyone was telling me my baby had reflux because he was so windy and was arching his back every time he was put down, but we soon figured out that if we didn't put him down he stopped arching. It helped us realise what was actually going on.'*

Conclusion

So, in a nutshell: a lot of babies have reflux, and overwhelmingly it's normal. When it becomes more tricky is if they are having unsettled behaviours, and you're trying to unpick whether it's to do with reflux, or something else.

I'd really encourage you to get along to a support group, and to see a breastfeeding counsellor or IBCLC, if at all possible, to help you work out what's going on for you, and how best to move forward. But it can be incredibly hard and emotional trying to cope with it all, especially if you're also trying to do a bit of detective work about what might be going on! And yet, no matter what's happening, keeping your baby close, and getting support for you is going to be key. Because you are doing *brilliantly*, but everyone needs help sometimes.

Sarah's story

My first pregnancy did not go at all to plan, due to pre-eclampsia. An early induction was needed and, ultimately, a C-section under general anaesthetic. I was then taken to a private room to recover, after a brief hello with my little girl (I was very groggy) before she was taken to SCBU, having been born premature and only 5lbs, where she was given a bottle. I really wanted to breastfeed, though, and was so disappointed that the opportunity might have already been lost.

As I lay there getting my head around what had happened, feeling sore and in shock, I felt such a sense of disappointment all round, especially as I hadn't yet held my baby. But during the night a midwife crept in with my baby in her arms. She said she needed to see her mum and to be fed. She put her into my arms and at last I could meet her properly. It was love at first sight.

The midwife was wonderful, understanding my discomfort and helping me to sit up and protect my wound with pillows to latch her on. With some adjustment, to my delight my baby started to suck and I felt an overwhelming sense of relief to hear her gulping. The midwife left me to it and, when she came back, put her into the crib by my bed, saying I could keep her. I lay on my side with the help of pillows, just gazing at her.

Later, at home, I was surrounded by family who had never breastfed and, although encouraging and loving, there was a sense that managing to breastfeed was luck and it probably wouldn't last. I had just moved to the area and didn't know many people, but thankfully had joined the NCT, which held regular new mums coffee mornings with trained breastfeeding counsellors. Those sessions were invaluable in keeping me going and an opportunity to talk to others about what was 'normal'.

Breastfeeding was something I was determined to do, but I constantly worried I was feeding her too much as she was always hungry. The best advice actually came from my grandmother-in-law. Now ninety, she had breastfed when her children had been born, as everyone did then. She came to stay and said, 'That baby is hungry.' She told me to relax, listen to my baby, and not watch the clock. It worked, and we got into a bit of a routine, but mostly for the first three months we just fed!

I loved breastfeeding so much. It became my time with my little girl and we continued for twelve months. I felt such satisfaction that this tiny baby grew so fast on my milk, and although the birth may not have gone to plan, I had nurtured her through. I am so proud of that.

10

Colic, wind and difficult evenings

OMG, we are *obsessed* with wind and babies! It's a major topic of conversation in support groups, online, from family and friends, and from health professionals too. I've devoted a whole chapter to this because I think it's really useful to break it all down and get a good understanding of what different terms mean, the products and treatments available, and what else might be happening.

What is colic?

Well, that depends who you're talking to, because, confusingly, this is one of those terms that's used in a variety of ways. Some people, for example, say colic to mean wind. Others say colic to mean unsettled behaviours. Some use it to mean crying in the evening.

The medical definition of colic is a baby that cries for at least three hours a day, at least three times a week, for at least three weeks. So it's not a diagnosis, so much as a description for a distressed baby. Why they're upset is frequently put down to wind, and it's common for these hours of upset to be in the evening, so I think that's why these terms get mixed up. But let's explore a bit more.

Babies that are crying for several hours at a time and on lots of occasions shouldn't be just dismissed as having colic. Colic is a definition not a diagnosis, and, generally speaking, isn't all that helpful to anyone. If your baby is crying a lot, something is wrong, and it can almost always be sorted.

It could be a feeding issue, it could be illness, it could be an allergy, or something else. But, sadly, babies often get labelled as having colic, and then nothing further is done about it. If you have concerns about your baby being unsettled or distressed, keep asking for help, and keep asking why. Have a look at the chapters on allergies, and reflux, which may help you unpick this too.

> 'She was such a screamy baby, constantly miserable and crying if she wasn't feeding. I knew something was wrong but kept getting told it was just colic and it would pass by the time she was three months old. There was no way I could keep going until three months, though, so I saw a lactation consultant, who picked up that she was showing lots of signs of allergy. I gave up dairy and, within a few days, she was like a different baby' – Vicky, mum to India.

Wind

On the one hand, it seems that every upset and all unsettled behaviour is attributed to wind, but, on the other, parents are still often told that you don't need to wind a breastfed baby. It's no wonder we feel so confused and out of depth with a new baby.

So *do* you need to wind a breastfed baby? Some, yes, some, no! Everybody is different, every baby is different, and whether they get wind or not will depend on lots of factors. As a general rule, try winding them after feeds (and/or between swapping boobs) and, as you get to know them over the weeks and months, you'll start to figure out what's right for them. Remember: so much about life with a new baby is getting to know them and building confidence in yourself.

What causes wind?

If getting feeding established is tricky (as it often is!), it may be that there is latching on and off, a bit of crying here and there and a bit of readjusting when milk starts to flow, and that can all lead to air being swallowed. And if your baby has a tongue tie, the restricted motion of the tongue can also cause more air to be swallowed. If you have a very fast flow of milk, or oversupply (too much milk), this can have an impact too.

Basically, the main cause of wind is to do with the actual action of feeding, but there will also be some wind that comes from the digestion of milk too. What you yourself eat and drink does *not* cause wind, though, unless your baby has an allergy to that food. If you eat lots of sprouts at Christmas, your baby won't get windy because of them. Your milk is made from your bloodstream, not your stomach contents. So you don't need to avoid onions or garlic, or any other foods that seem to get randomly mentioned when parents report they're struggling.

Similarly, if you drink fizzy drinks, they won't make your baby windy either, as it's *your* body dealing with the bubbles, not theirs. And gas that comes from the bottom end? Well, that's usually from the digestive process. Just a natural waste product.

How will I know they've got wind?

Well, you might not – honestly! You'll know something's up, but, in the early days, it's usually a process of elimination, literally going through a checklist at times. If they're not conked out asleep, then they're likely to be signalling for something, either by rooting and squirming around, or whinging and crying. You'll spend quite a lot of time wondering what might be up and trying to figure it out, and that's completely normal.

Remember: babies want to spend a huge amount of time latched on, and so, when they're not, they will often wriggle and moan and try to make their way back there asap. But because they've not long fed, it's common for us to assume it can't be that they want to feed, so we start to wonder if perhaps it's wind. So we pat and rub their back, and they get increasingly distressed because they're not latched back on, and we figure the wind must be pretty bad, as it's not coming up and they're getting pretty upset . . . Eventually, after some crying and distress all round, a burp comes up, but, in actual fact, it's because all that crying has caused a load of air in their belly. But, of course, we don't know that, and we feel very satisfied that after a long time of trying that stubborn wind has finally come up. So we get stuck in a mindset that our baby gets bad trapped wind, and with every episode where we wind them and no burps arrive, it secures the theory further.

However, if we'd just latched them on to test what was needed, probably all that would have been avoided. So, first port of call: always offer the boob where you can. Because if a burp doesn't come up in the first minute or two, it's because there isn't one, and they need something else. So please don't feel you have to spend hours patting and rubbing and doing 'bicycle legs'. All that's generally needed is to hold them close to your body, leaning

Wonky winding

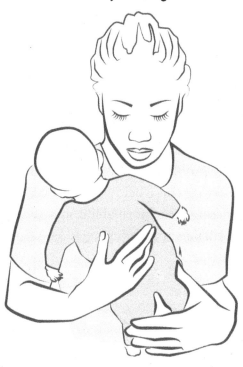

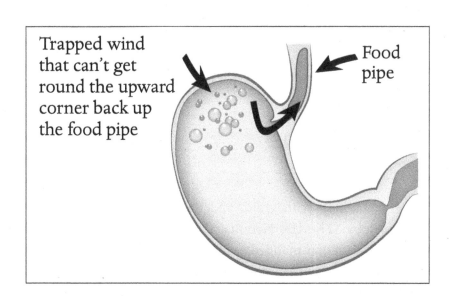

Trapped wind that can't get round the upward corner back up the food pipe

Food pipe

over toward their left side slightly, as this supports the air release using the natural anatomy of their stomach and windpipe.

Is all crying abnormal?

Babies *do* cry, of course. I'm not suggesting that all crying is abnormal. And some babies cry more than others. But for the most part, if we meet their need, the crying will calm. Crying only becomes a problem when we can't stop it, and/or it's excessive. The crying curve below gives us an idea of how much babies may cry as a part of normal life, and also a helpful look at how thing can change at differing ages.

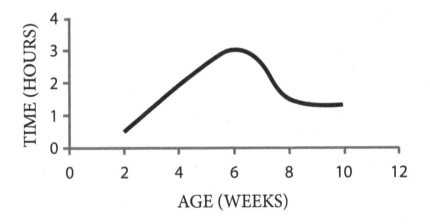

Do colic drops help?

Short answer: no.

They don't help with wind, and they don't help babies that are unhappy. The UK National Guidance suggests that these shouldn't be recommended, and I would agree. Not only does the evidence show they don't work, but they don't help to get to the underlying cause of the issue. Some people do feel that colic drops helped their baby with wind, though, and there's a reason why. Do you remember in science class at school how they got you to do the experiment where you add bicarbonate of soda to vinegar and watch all the gas bubbles come up? Well, that's basically what's happening with colic drops: we're adding a substance to the baby's stomach acid that gathers up those air bubbles and then: voila! A burp! Then we think, 'I gave colic drops, the baby burped.' But, actually, it's 'I gave colic drops, it caused wind, the baby burped it up'!

Don't waste your money on drops; buy yourself a treat instead, because it's hard work looking after an unsettled baby, or any baby!

What about difficult evenings?

Late afternoon and evenings with a baby can be, well . . . challenging. To put it politely! And this seems to be one of the reasons the term colic gets brought up so much for this time of day.

Let me describe what can happen in this time, and what might be going on.

A large percentage of babies seem to change at this time: they change their feeding frequency, their feeding behaviours, and even their temperament. They often want to feed almost non-stop too, and yet when they do they get frustrated and upset. Pulling on and off, crying at the breast, tugging and hitting, even pushing away despite showing feeding cues is common. It feels like you can't please them or satisfy them, even though you're responding to their cues. They're fussy and cranky and even plain old upset and crying. It can feel like they're rejecting you, and it's horrible. They seem like they're tired, but when they sleep it's for a few minutes before they're up again. All this and you often feel like your boobs are deflated air socks flapping in the breeze. Rest assured this is really common; hard, but common.

So what's going on? Well, it's partly to do with those pesky hormones I'm afraid. We know that hormones fluctuate over the 24 hours, and it seems that late afternoon/evening time is a particularly difficult period. This leads to milk supply running not lower, but seemingly slower. Breasts often feel soft and empty, and this can be really unnerving for parents, especially when their baby is getting pretty peeved off at the breast, or wanting to be there relentlessly. It can add to that nagging feeling of 'I don't have enough milk'. But breasts are never empty, and milk production continues 24/7. It's just this weird time of day when it all goes a bit mad.

The behaviours that babies exhibit at this time are stimulation behaviours. A little like kittens knead at the breast to encourage milk flow, human babies pad and fist the breast too, but also tug around, come on and off, squirm and fuss (you'll notice these behaviours during growth spurts too – all messages of 'I need more milk to flow please!').

Because feeding can be so difficult at this time, parents often resort back to that ingrained underlying message of 'the baby doesn't need feeding' and assume something else must be going on. What doesn't help is that this hormonal change not only seems to affect us physically, but emotionally too. Tearful, irritable, vulnerable, paranoid . . . a range of negative feelings seem to hit hard. Whenever I talk about this with new parents,

I see an absolute lightbulb moment happen in their face, often followed by the words 'I'm so glad it's not just me' or 'that explains so much', even sometimes tears of relief.

Another phenomenon that ignites the same spark of recognition is the 'Bed Dread'. As the day heads towards the night, no matter how well you've been feeling during the day, fear about the night starts to set in. A feeling of 'I can't do it, please don't make me do it' seems to loom over us. It's common to feel quite resentful at this point too.

During the early weeks, a massive amount of changes occur, and babies' brains are developing seriously fast. As they spend more time waking up to the world and alert, they're taking on board a huge amount of stimulation. Noises, sights, smells, feelings: there's a huge amount going on and it's a lot for them to process. By the time you get to the evening, they're absolutely wired. If you've ever experienced multi-sensory overload, try to remember that feeling and then maybe you can better understand why babies are pretty cranky by the end of the day.

As with a lot of these things, however, this can't necessarily be solved simply, but having knowledge about what's going on, that it's normal, and that you're not alone, can help enormously.

So, what can you do to help? Firstly: try to plan things so you head towards the late afternoon having eaten and drunk plenty. You definitely don't want to veer into 'hangry' territory, so make sure you have easily grabbable one-handed snacks dotted around the place.

Make sure baby has had plenty of sleep during the day. This is often at the breast, but any other way that they sleep is fine too. If you can manage a sleep during the day too, that's fantastic as well. And, as ever, skin-to-skin cuddles with baby can really help calm you both, while co-bathing can be lovely and soothing too.

Another key tip is to get, and use, a sling. Not just in the evening but during the day too. That closeness and comfort will help support them to rest and relax, which can lead to an easier evening.

Then, above all, offer the breast frequently, and try not to worry if they are unsettled when they're there. But don't assume that if they rejected it ten minutes ago that they don't want it now. They can be really fickle in the evening.

And reach out for support. Family, friends, a postnatal doula . . . anyone who can help you out with whatever you might need. In my experience, these difficulties often start around Week 2–3, and peak around Week 6-8, before gradually starting to ease.

So, if you're having difficult evenings, it may be a typical, though hard, part of new baby life. But if you have any worries at all, a breastfeeding counsellor or lactation consultant (IBCLC) would be a great person to speak to. An understanding of what's going on can make *such* a huge difference, and there's usually some adjustments to feeding that can help too. Or it may be that what's going on won't seem normal to them, and, if so, they will then be on hand to help you figure out what else might be happening.

> 'Oh, gosh, I used to absolutely dread the evenings. It was like someone had swapped my baby for someone else's. He was so grumpy, and feeding was difficult, and it made me feel like I was a complete failure as a mum. Speaking to my baby group friends helped as it was happening to a lot of them too, and it did pass after a while.'

Conclusion

Young babies cry, and have a lot of needs, and it can be pretty hard at times. Usually it's normal, but if you're finding that you're having a lot of times where you can't stop the crying, it's a sign to seek some help. Getting some feeding support is a good place to start, and some practical support for you is also going to be really helpful too. And as you learn to get to know your baby, and know yourself as a parent, things *will* get easier. You'll learn to trust your instincts too.

Oh, and know this: 'You'll just know what their different cries mean' is most definitely *not* true for most of us! You'll learn, sure, but it takes time. Be patient with yourself.

Lisa's story

Thrush: it was awful, and I was trying to look after a three-year-old, so I just got on with it. I didn't really understand what was wrong and, in a sleep-deprived haze, I just carried on with the day to day. My baby's constant crying meant I didn't want to be around people, let alone mother-and-baby groups. It seems obvious now, as I write this, that I was in a really bad place and should've asked for help, but that's the problem. When you are in a bad place, it's so easy to close the door on everyone and everything and just cuddle your baby and look after a toddler in the safe space of your own home. I felt like everyone around me was having blissful experiences, and then there was me, with a child who cried solidly for three months. Breastfeeding then became another problem. I had never found it particularly easy with my first son, but this was harder. Bottles became the easy solution that I could swap to. I had no clue what was wrong with me. I just made decisions on my own, based on zero medical facts, in the hope it would go away. I didn't have the capacity to persevere or seek help. I was wrong to not reach out. When I finally got help, the problem was easy to fix, but, sadly, I'd given up breastfeeding and had mentally moved on from even wanting to breastfeed. The health visitor explained what my baby and I had, and I felt so guilty about this and angry at myself for not seeking help sooner. Yay! More mum guilt! The health visitor was so lovely. She even reassured me that the time I had breast-fed my son had done him good and that I should be proud of myself. It was what I needed to hear. I wish I'd sought help earlier instead of just getting on with it. If you are showing symptoms, please don't leave it like I did. Reach out to friends, and most definitely a midwife or health professional.

11

Allergies and the breastfed baby

A common and increasingly popular suggestion in the breast-feeding world is that parents cut out dairy from their diet, to help with any number of baby problems, from wind, to vomiting, to sleep. In fact, I'm not sure I've come across a parent in the last few years that hasn't had this suggested to them by someone! But, on the other hand, you've got parents being told allergies can't even exist in breastfed babies. It's all *very* confusing! But this chapter is going to guide you through the noise, and help you work out whether you really need to be giving up dairy, or anything else, for that matter.

Can breastfed babies have allergies?

Yes, they certainly can; they are just mini humans, after all. And it seems that rates of allergies are increasing. Unfortunately, as with a lot of things breastfeeding-related, we just don't have as much research as we need into this area. However, it's believed that up to 5–10 per cent of babies may have allergies, and studies also show that this is more likely to be the case if the baby has had any infant formula, and/or if there are allergies in their parent/s or sibling/s.

The most common allergy in the under fives is to cow's milk. However, just like adults, babies can actually be allergic to any food. There are some that are much more likely: eggs, peanuts, wheat, fish and soya are all common allergens.

How do I know if my baby has an allergy?

Symptoms of allergy in babies can also be signs of lots of other things as well, and, of course, it's possible to have other issues going on at the same time as allergies too. It can be really hard to figure out *what's* going on! (or even if it's just normal). As with most things, an IBCLC can help you if you're struggling to get to the bottom of what might be happening.

Two of the most common signs of allergy, however, are unusual poos, and skin problems. Breastfed baby poo should be, on the whole, soft, a yellowy colour, and may have some seedy-looking bits in it. Baby poo is sometimes described as being like runny peanut butter, or wholegrain mustard (hope you're not eating your tea while reading this!).

Babies with an allergy, though, often have digestive issues, which show up in their poo. Poo may be green, mucous-y, smelly, excessive in frequency, or have blood in it (sometimes this is just a speck here or there).* Skin issues, meanwhile, can include eczema, frequent nappy rash, and cradle cap.

There are many other symptoms too, including:

- Tummy pains and excessive wind

- Congested nose and stuffy breathing

- Vomiting

---

* If your baby ever passes blood, please get them checked over promptly by a
  medical professional.

- Weight gain problems

- Hiccupping

- Sneezing

- Feeding problems

- Sweating

- Unsettled and unhappy behaviours

As mentioned, a lot of these symptoms can also be signs of other things too, and I think that's why we've got lots of allergies being missed, but also lots of allergies being misdiagnosed when they are actually something else.

So, because it can involve a bit of detective work to find out what's happening, if you're unsure, I'd strongly encourage you to try to work with someone, ideally (you guessed it) an IBCLC, to help figure this stuff out. It will set you on the quickest, easiest route to getting things sorted, though it still may not be easy, I'm afraid. You might be able to get a referral to the infant feeding team via your local NHS trust, or some parents choose to work privately with someone if they can't get access to any support for free.

Can you get tests for allergies?

This is where it gets a little tricky. There are two types of allergy, IgE, and Non IgE. IgE tend to be more immediate reactions, while Non IgE are more delayed and reactions happen over the following day or so.

IgE allergies can be tested for, using skin prick tests. But there are no tests for Non IgE allergies, which is difficult. The way to figure out if there is a Non IgE allergy (which also works for IgE, by the way) is by removing the suspected allergen from your diet and seeing if symptoms improve. In order for it to be diagnosed formally, you're then meant to remove this allergen for at least two weeks, then add it back in and find out whether symptoms return, before removing it again. This then clearly shows it's the cause of the symptoms.

In my experience, a lot of parents don't add the allergen back in again, though, as sometimes the difference is so remarkable, and the improvement so drastic, that they are reluctant to go back to how things were, which is completely understandable, I think!

Years ago, we were told you needed to remove the allergen for at least six weeks for it to be fully out of your diet, but actually this isn't the case at all. In fact, it will be out of your system pretty quickly, within 24 hours. But the inflammation to the body that it's caused can last longer and reactions can go on for several days. You will usually know within a few days to a week if you've found the allergen that's causing problems (though sometimes there is more than one, of course, which can cause it to take longer).

How do I know which allergen it might be?

So, you've worked out that your baby has a lot of symptoms of allergy, and you've worked through some of the other things it might be instead, but so far there's no (or minimal) improvement. Now you want to try to remove whatever the allergen may be from your diet to help them, but how do you know what to remove?

A really helpful starting point is keeping a food and symptom diary. Note down every day what you've had to eat and drink, including any medications or supplements. You can also write how things have been that day, how feeds have been, what nappies have been like, how your baby's skin is, temperament, essentially whatever symptoms might be relevant to your situation. Looking back over previous days and weeks, you may then be able to start to notice a pattern – for example, every time you have an egg, over the next couple of days symptoms increase. It's also worth thinking about what you consume a lot of, and checking through any allergies or intolerances going back through both families, as these are more likely to be an issue.

If you can't notice a pattern, some people choose to eliminate one of the top offenders, such as dairy, and see how things go. If you see improvement, fantastic. If not, you can move on to a different food. Some parents choose to eliminate more than one thing at a time, which is fine, but difficult. It might calm the symptoms sooner, though, because you're more likely to be cutting out the problem. But you then need to discover which one of those things was causing an issue, by slowly reintroducing things one at a time every few days or so, and this may mean you're on a restricted diet for longer.

For some people, that's okay, as they want to get to the root of the problem quickly; for others, it really is too hard to do so much at once, and I totally get that. An elimination diet can be pretty tough, especially when you're looking after a baby, and a baby that's having difficulties too, so try to take any shortcuts that you can, for example ready meals, and accept help if it's offered. If someone wants to go ahead and cook you that dairy-free, egg-free, peanut-free dinner, say yes!

Remember, though, if you're removing things from your diet, you need to think about how you'll get the vitamins and nutrients you need. For example, if you remove dairy, it's recommended to take a calcium supplement. Your baby won't need anything else, however, as your milk will still contain everything they need. (NB: In the UK, it's recommended that babies take a daily Vitamin D supplement.)

Don't forget that if you do remove a food, it does need to be in its entirety. Sometimes foods are in things we wouldn't expect, like milk in some crisps, for example, so be careful to read the back of packets and watch for any sneaky ingredients getting in.

I've found the food causing the problem, what do I do now?

Ask your GP for a referral to dieticians for help moving forward. This will include what needs replacing in your diet, but also how best to get your baby started on solid food when the time comes (known as weaning). There is no need to start solids early for a baby with allergies. Weaning is mostly beyond the scope of this book, but I would always advise in general that you should wait for signs of readiness (see p.270) and I've recommended some other resources on p. 276.

If my baby can't tolerate dairy, can I have lactose-free milk instead?

Unfortunately not. The baby is reacting to the protein in cow's milk, not the lactose. Lactose is in all milk, and is actually the main sugar in your breastmilk! And babies don't have a problem with lactose the way adults might. As we grow older, our need for milk diminishes and so does our ability to digest it. This is why adults may struggle with dairy intolerance as they get older.

192

There are some problems that babies can have with milk sugars, though, but these are different to adult intolerance. One is called Galactocaemia. This is an incredibly rare and serious condition (affecting about 1 in every 40,000 babies) that will become apparent in the first few days of life. The other is a type of lactose intolerance, but with different symptoms than those seen in adults.

You may not be aware that the composition of your milk changes, from feed to feed and day by day: breastmilk is perfect in its design. On the odd occasion, however – for example, if your baby has been unwell with a tummy bug – their body's ability to break down lactose can temporarily be reduced. Usually this will cause a large amount of green poo, often explosive, lots of wind, and often an unhappy baby too. This is called secondary lactose intolerance. It will resolve itself in time, and you don't need to change to any specialist milks; continuing to breastfeed is great.

Another time lactose intolerance may be an issue is if you have too much milk. The amount of lactose your baby gets may be too high for their body to process, not because they have an intolerance, but just because it's just too much to handle. The symptoms will be the same as above. If you think you have an oversupply, do seek support, as there are things that can be done to help. But, above all, please try not to worry about lactose, and remember that it's cow's milk protein that causes the allergy.

Would it be better to stop breastfeeding if my baby has an allergy?

This is so hard. I know how difficult breastfeeding a baby that has an allergy can be, and you may be wondering if it would be better to just stop and move on to formula. I would say that for some people it may be.

However, it's important to remind ourselves that parents who felt they *had* to stop breastfeeding often feel regretful, and may experience a sense of loss even amounting to grief that their journey didn't go the way they had planned. So while feeding a baby who has an allergy is really tough, think carefully about your feelings, and try not to make big decisions on a bad day. When it comes to your baby, it's great for them if you can continue breastfeeding and keep yourself well while managing the allergy, despite the challenges.

My doctor has suggested a special formula milk?

Sometimes families that have a baby with allergies may find their doctor recommends a specialist type of formula milk to use instead of breastfeeding. This may be due to concerns that an elimination diet may be difficult or unhealthy for you, or a misunderstanding that breastmilk might in some way be lacking if you remove things from your diet.

However, there's no evidence that special formulas are better for a baby with allergies than breastmilk. Our milk contains a lot more than calories, fats, vitamins and minerals. There are incredible things in breastmilk that have not been replicated in any formulas, such as hormones and immune factors. And, of course, breastfeeding is about so much more than just milk – it's comfort, bonding, sleep support and so much more.

So, there's absolutely no reason to switch to formula milk if you don't want to. The Academy of Breastfeeding Medicine (ABM) has a protocol about allergy and breastfeeding that may be useful for your doctor.

I thought breastfeeding was meant to prevent allergies?

If you put two large groups of babies in a room – one group breastfed, one not – the breastfed group would have less babies with allergies in. So breastfeeding doesn't *prevent* allergies, per se, but they're less likely. It can feel like a real slap in the face when you've worked so hard to breastfeed, and then found that your baby has allergies anyway. But please know that breastfeed-ing is still so beneficial to them, and all the hard work you've done and continue to do is not for nothing. You really are doing such an amazing job.

Conclusion

Lots of parents are advised to remove dairy, or other foods, from their diet to see if it helps with a variety of symptoms. Often this isn't needed and there are other things going on, such as feeding issues, or a need for support with baby's normal but tricky behaviours (like wanting to be held 24/7!). Sometimes, though, babies do have allergies, and figuring out what they are can be complicated. Working with someone experienced in infant feeding and allergies can be really beneficial: you don't have to do it alone.

Lucy's story

My second baby took a while to conceive, and my older daughter was three when she was born. Breastfeeding my first baby had been challenging and scary at times, but, on the whole, pretty straightforward; she was a premature, small baby and, needing to catch up, a hungry feeder. Once I had accepted it was *okay* to devote myself to feeding her whenever she asked (constantly, it seemed!), we got it down to a fine art, and feeding became one of life's great pleasures for twelve months.

When my second baby arrived, I expected to latch her on and never look back . . . I was so wrong. No one had warned me that every baby is different.

Although my second daughter was premature too, she didn't feed in the same way at all. She wasn't a fussy feeder, but moved about a lot, hardly ever still even when glugging away.

With my first baby, in the early mornings we were both ready for a good long feed, her for hunger, me for relief from discomfort due to having lots of milk in the mornings. Second baby wasn't bothered, really, until later on, so it was a struggle for me to manage and quite painful at times. Someone suggested expressing, but that, of course, just produced more milk.

I sometimes used to wake her in the night (I know!), so that she could sleepily feed and I wouldn't be so engorged first thing. Not an ideal solution, as, like all new parents, I was desperate for sleep.

By around two months, my breasts were not so full and we had got into some sort of pattern: I had an early cuppa and a couple of biscuits with my toddler until no. 2 was ready to feed. Things settled down and we fed for twelve months. Not quite as relaxing as my first baby, as this one was a wriggler and distracted by anything, especially watching her big sister, so feeding often had to be in a quiet place. Despite all that, I just loved breastfeeding her. To watch her grow into a chubby, happy baby was so fulfilling and we enjoyed our quiet times with her little starfish hands pushing at my breasts like a kitten!

12
Tongue tie

Tongue ties get blamed for a whole lot of problems, and there still seems to be a lot of misinformation about them. Sometimes it seems that *every* baby has one, other times that parents are told they don't even exist! Well, they certainly exist, but, yes, they can be over-diagnosed too, so I want to give you some information in this chapter so that you can feel more confident navigating through this area, if you need to.

What is tongue tie?

If you stick out your tongue and lift it up, you might see there's a little stringy bit connecting the tongue to the floor of the mouth: this is called the lingual frenulum. This frenulum is different in everyone, just as our ears and noses are different to each other; we all have different anatomies, after all. In some people it's long, some short, some thin, some thick, stretchy or not, far back, far forward . . . it can vary a lot. In some people, though, this frenulum may be causing some restriction to how the tongue moves around, and this is when it gets termed a 'tongue tie'. It's thought to affect up to 1 in 10 babies.

It might be that the frenulum is too short, too far forward, too stiff, or a combination. The key is that it's not really about how it looks, it's about how it impacts on the tongue's function. People are often aware of the frenulum attaching right at the very tip of the tongue as being a tongue tie, and, of course, this may be the case, but if it's very long and stretchy, the tongue may have no problem at all moving around. Equally, the frenulum may be quite far back under the tongue, but if it's very short and doesn't stretch, it may have a big effect on restricting tongue movement. It's not just a straightforward, obvious thing sometimes, and it needs careful, experienced assessment.

Who can check for tongue tie and how do they check?

Unfortunately, not every health professional you come into contact with will be able to assess for tongue tie. Even in an infant feeding team, there may only be one or two people who know how to diagnose it. Tongue tie checks are not a routine part of care, so don't assume your baby has or will be checked; you may need to seek out specialist help.

In order to assess for a tie, the assessor will have a gloved finger, or fingers, in the baby's mouth feeling and checking a wide range of tongue movements and functions and it will usually take several minutes. It should also include taking of a full history, and observing a full feed. It is not just a case of looking in the baby's mouth.

There is a commonly accepted myth that only a frenulum very visibly right at the tip of the tongue is a tie, so parents are often told their baby doesn't have a tie because someone has just looked and assumed all is well. Which is why the very first thing I ask a parent that is having struggles, and tells me their baby has been checked for tongue tie, is: did the person put gloved fingers in their mouth? If not, I know that we still need to assess. You *cannot* tell if there is a tie just by looking.

So, who can do this assessment? That's going to vary based on where you are. There is no set person, or qualification, for tongue tie assessment. Even as IBCLCs, not all of us are trained. However, those who *are* trained will always also be registered health professionals. Often the best thing to do is to ask your midwife or health visitor to refer your baby to the infant feeding team or tongue tie service. There are private services, too.

If you do seek someone privately, try to work with someone who has breastfeeding knowledge as well, like an IBCLC or breastfeeding counsellor.

> 'I'd asked a few times if my baby had tongue tie as I'd read about it and really felt it fit with what we were experiencing, but I kept getting told no because Emily looked fine and she could stick her tongue out. It was weeks before I got referred to the infant feeding team, who recognised straight away that she had a tongue tie and snipped it there and then. Things were so much better after that'– Anna, mum to Emily.

What are the signs?

What might show that baby has a tie? How do you even know if you need an assessment?

The restriction in each baby's tongue will be different, and affect feeding in a different way. Some will be way more obvious than others. But I'd say, if in doubt, get the ball rolling and get yourself referred. In some places it can take some time to get seen, and it's better to get on the waiting list, and find you don't need the appointment, than the other way around. Specifically, though, some signs of a tongue tie can be:

- Painful feeds (nipple and breast)
- Misshapen nipples after feeds
- Vasospasm
- Latching difficulties
- Slipping back or off during feeds
- Weight gain and/or milk supply issues
- Long feeds
- Short feeds
- Very frequent feeds
- Infrequent pooing
- Blocked ducts and mastitis
- Lip blisters
- Clicking noise during feeds
- Unsettled baby
- Wind
- Reflux

It's so important to mention that *all* of these things can also be absolutely nothing to do with tongue tie at all. However, the opposite is also true and it may be that you have loads of these symptoms and they've all been attributed to something else but are actually because of a tie. This is why it's really important to work with someone who understands breastfeeding, tongue ties, and infant behaviours.

Even if there is a tie, there are very often adjustments that can be made to improve things, even if they don't resolve them completely. So if you know your baby has a tie and you're waiting for treatment, please don't stop asking for support and working toward changes.

> *'Bobby had his tie snipped but it didn't make much difference. It wasn't until I started lying down to feed with him on my tummy that our latch sorted itself out and it didn't hurt anymore'*– Reni, mum to Bobby.

What's the treatment for tongue tie?

The person who assesses your baby should be able to discuss with you whether they think it would be beneficial to leave the tie, treat it, or wait a while and reassess the situation. And the choice is always yours. They can give you recommendations, but it's your baby, your feeding journey, and it's up to you what decision you make.

Sometimes, you may be working on making some changes to feeding – for example, the way your baby positions and latches at the breast – and it's recommended that you wait and see if these improve the problems before going ahead with treatment for the tie. Which makes complete sense, really, especially if it's early on in their life.

Other times, you may be advised that the tie is best treated straight away. And often it can be done there and then. The procedure itself is actually quite straightforward (so much so that private practitioners can do this in your home).

The baby usually gets swaddled to keep them still, and for comfort, and their head will be held gently still. The frenulum under the tongue is stretched using the practitioner's fingers, and then quickly snipped/divided with sterile blunt ended scissors (or sometimes a laser, though this isn't common in the UK). It often pings apart a little, like if you snipped through a stretched elastic band. It takes a matter of seconds, and then they're unwrapped and handed to you.

These simple steps give immediate release to the tongue, which is then able to move around more freely. However, the baby will have to learn how to use their newly freed tongue and strengthen muscles in different ways. So while sometimes feeds are immediately better, sometimes it can take a bit of time over the following days or weeks.

The procedure is usually done without anaesthetic, partly because the anaesthetic injection itself would be more painful than the division (if you've ever had local anaesthetic at the dentist, you'll know it's really sore!). It's also because we really don't want to numb up babies' tongues when they need and want to feed so frequently. We usually do the division and then offer the baby the breast immediately (literally seconds after). It helps calm and soothe them if they've found it painful. Almost every baby is quite happy once they've had a feed. Though, in fact, some babies sleep through it! Some babies, however, will be a bit uncomfy for a day or two, but frequent feeds and skin-to-skin cuddles help.

Does snipping tongue tie help? Yes, it certainly can, and for some parents and babies it can be life changing. For others, they find the procedure doesn't help as much as they would hope. I suspect that this is because the problems they were having were attributed to the tie, when in fact they were down to something else that wasn't rectified. This is why it's so very important that a tongue tie snip isn't done in isolation. Breastfeeding support and manage-ment is crucial in making things better.

It can be a big decision to decide whether to have your baby's tie divided, and, as parents, our instincts are to protect our babies from pain and upset, so we can feel a lot of emotions about this. If worries about the procedure are bothering you, try to keep in mind that it's usually very quick. I've divided hundreds of ties, and I'd say over 90 per cent of parents said the words 'Oh, was that it?' as I handed their baby back to them!

> 'The midwife was so helpful. She showed us what was going on with his tongue and the problems it could be causing, and then talked through what we could do and how they would divide it. We decided to have it divided and it was done quickly right then. He was upset for a few minutes, but after a feed he was fine. The benefit of doing it definitely outweighed the negatives.' – Cara, parent to Idris.

Aftercare after division

There will often be a little bleeding during the tongue tie snip, but once the baby has fed, this should stop and no further bleeding is expected. As with any wound on the body there is a small chance of infection, but the chances are very small. There is lots of lovely breastmilk helping keep infection away and helping it heal, after all. But there will be a diamond-shaped ulcer under-neath the tongue, that will turn a white, cream or yellow in colour, and it may stay there for a couple of weeks.

The practitioner you work with will explain to you what aftercare they recommend. In the past, some practitioners have recom-mended wound massage, though most have now moved away from this, as it's been found to be of minimal benefit and quite distressing to parents and baby. All practitioners should encourage breastfeeding support as a minimum level of aftercare. Some may also suggest bodywork, which is discussed below.

Can tongue ties reattach or regrow?

I've mentioned several times throughout this book that we just don't have as much research into breastfeeding issues as we should and tongue tie, unfortunately, is another one of those areas. Different practitioners have different thoughts on whether tongue ties can reattach or regrow. Some argue that there can be growth of the frenulum after it's been divided, some suspect it's that the frenulum wasn't divided fully.

Either way, if the restricted tongue movement is still causing you and your baby problems, it can, on occasion, require a second division of the frenulum. My advice would be, as above, that you absolutely must work with someone to look fully at you, your baby, and breastfeeding as a whole to see what's happening.

Faux ties and bodywork

On occasion, babies may have signs of tongue movement restriction but these may not be caused by the frenulum. They can, instead, be due to tightness in the body. These have been termed 'faux ties' by well-respected tongue tie practitioner Alison Hazelbaker. Again, this is an area that's lacking in research, though I suspect it's something that's going to get a lot more interest in the future.

Anecdotally, parents often report that they've had much success with approaches commonly referred to as 'bodywork', such as cranial osteopathy, both for problems like faux ties that are causing a direct feeding problem, but also issues like torticollis – muscle tightness or shortening in one side of the neck that may be causing problems indirectly.

What about lip ties?

In some countries, it is believed that the upper lip frenulum can interfere with feeding for some babies too, and so needs to be divided if there are feeding issues. However, arguably the evidence isn't there to support this.

It is normal anatomy to have a frenulum under your top lip, just as it is under your tongue. But the difference is that the tongue is a vital collection of muscles that are greatly involved with breastfeeding, whereas the top lip needs to simply remain neutral. With a deep, asymmetric, effective latch, the top lip will *not* be turned up like 'fish lips' or 'pringle' lips. The bottom lip will be turned out wide, but the top lip will be in a neutral or slightly everted position.

In fact, if the top lip is having to grip on to the breast (which often causes a lip blister), this suggests there is a problem with the latch, but that's not due to the lip frenulum, and correcting the problem will also correct the lip gripping. This may be down to the way the baby is positioned and brought onto the breast, a tongue tie, or something like torticollis, that I've mentioned above.

Conclusion

Information about tongue ties has been mixed over the years, and although things are improving, you can still come across mixed messages and differing opinions. Don't be embarrassed to ask the person working with you about their experience or training in tongue ties, as they'll be very happy to tell you if they're appropriately qualified. It's important that you get good care: you *deserve* good care.

Faye's story

When I became pregnant with my first baby, I was so excited to be a mum, and, honestly, I never really thought about how I was going to feed her, whether that be breastfeed, combination feed or formula feed.

At one of my midwife appointments, my midwife asked how I was planning on feeding my baby. I instantly replied breastfeeding, and thought I'd breastfeed for around six weeks. Oh, how wrong I was!

When my baby was born (induction in a hospital setting), she was placed on my chest and instantly began to do the 'breast crawl' and latched herself on! It honestly felt a bit strange, but wasn't painful or uncomfortable, thankfully. We were then discharged from hospital on Day 2, exclusively breastfeeding.

Nothing prepared me for Night 2, when baby was latching on and off all night. I felt really out of my depth and was so sleep deprived. I really questioned my choice to breastfeed at that point, if I'm honest. The community midwife came to weigh baby on Day 3 and she had an 8 per cent weight loss.

The midwife reassured me that this was within the normal range and to carry on breastfeeding on demand. I explained about the struggle I had the night before and the midwife provided lots of reassurance that this was normal and that I was doing a great job responding to my baby's needs. I had an infant feeding support worker visit me that afternoon, and she assessed latch and said that baby was slightly central on the breast, leading to a shallow latch. She showed me how to rectify this, and, basically, the rest is history!

I continued feeding on demand and baby maintained good weight gain and nappy output. I was happy and was beginning to gain confidence feeding outside the safety of our house. At my six-week health visitor check, I asked if I had to move baby on to bottles now, and the health visitor asked why. I explained that I thought people only breastfed for a few weeks. She explained that my breastmilk was tailored to my baby's needs and, unless I wanted to move to bottles, I could carry on breastfeeding for however long I and baby were happy to do so.

In the end, I fed my eldest until she was two years and four months old. In that time, I travelled to Thailand with my husband and daughter twice; I never had to worry about bringing formula with me or sterilising bottles etc and it really was so convenient for us and our lifestyle.

My breastfeeding journey with my son was a lot more difficult, but, thankfully, I knew I was capable of having a positive feeding journey and was able to successfully feed him. He's now three years and ten months old and still feeds occasionally.

Breastfeeding has truly changed my life and I am so thankful to be able to have had the support from my family and professionals to help me do this.

13

Myths

An interesting aspect of the breastfeeding world is that there are a lot of strange myths that just won't disappear! They can cause real damage to breastfeeding, in some cases, and most definitely make us worry about and question our abilities as a parent. There's a multitude of reasons why these exist, but, above all, it's that humans look for patterns, and when they find one, even if it's not correct, they stick with it, spread it, and then everyone believes it! It can be really hard to debunk these things once they get hold. But, I promise you, the things I outline below are just that: myths.

Foremilk/hindmilk

For a long time, we were told that there were two types of milk that were made by the breast: foremilk and hindmilk. The foremilk was the low fat, watery milk at the beginning of the feed; the hindmilk was the fatty milk at the end of the feed. But as we've learned more about breastfeeding and breastmilk, we've realised that these terms are misleading and unhelpful. The short version is: forget about it! But if you want to know more about why, I'll explain.

There aren't two types of milk made by the breast. Yes, there can be a change in the amount of fat as a breastfeed goes on, but it's gradual, doesn't happen at any set point or time, and isn't always the case! On a very simple level, the fat globules tend to be more sticky and take longer to dislodge and head down toward the nipple. So the beginning of the feed can be a little less fatty (though still fantastic milk!) and it gets more fatty as it goes along. However, it's not as straightforward as this, I'm afraid, and that it can vary due to a variety of factors, for example, when you last fed, or the time of day.

Imagine you're going to run a hot tap. When you first start it running, it starts cold and takes a bit of time for the hot to come through. If you run it again shortly after, the hot will be readily available, but if you leave it for a longer gap, there will be cold first before the hot. It's pretty much the same with breastmilk and fat content. If you've not long fed, it is likely to be higher in fat. This is why you don't need to worry about frequent feeds and fat content of milk.

The main message here is to just forget about the fat content and feed your baby when they need feeding, and for whatever reason. Your baby, and your body, know just what to do.

Keep the baby on the same side for X minutes

Another myth, that arises from the foremilk/hindmilk myth above, is that babies should stay on one breast for a certain amount of minutes, or to go back onto the same breast if they want to feed again within a certain time frame.

Now, this usually comes with the intention of getting more 'fatty milk', but we know from above it doesn't really work like that. Plus, weight gain is actually determined by the overall volume of milk taken in 24 hours, not by anything to do with specific fat composition.

Actually, by keeping the baby on the same breast, they tend to take *less* milk overall, which can lead to lower weight gain and, in turn, lower supply.

Let me explain: babies are driven by flow of milk, so when the milk ejection reflex happens, that's when they really start glugging away. By switching breasts, the stimulation on the second side causes more milk ejections, and therefore more drinking. This in turn leads to better weight gain and better supply (because remember: the more they take, the more you make!). Because they tend to drink less, keeping a baby on the one side for any length of time is actually a technique used for *reducing* supply! So it's definitely not something most people should do (if you do need to do this, it should be done with trained support, to reduce the risk of mastitis).

For most babies, let them feed from the first side until they come off and then offer the second. For those with weight gain or supply issues, encouraging frequent swaps is beneficial to get more drinking going on.

Routines

There is enormous pressure on families to get babies into routines, both for feeding and for sleep; to have them feeding at set intervals, sleeping for long periods, settling in their own sleep spaces. The pressure is so huge that we've even got to the point where we're actually worried something is wrong if we aren't managing to do this – wrong with the baby, or wrong with our parenting. That we're doing a bad job, or somehow failing them if they're not doing what they 'should be'.

But babies aren't meant to be in routines! Babies haven't read books that suggest they should feed, play, then sleep for certain time periods. Babies just have needs that need meeting, and they have no control on when those happen. Especially in the first few months, there really is often no pattern to anything, and that's completely normal!

Trying to stretch out gaps between feeds, or stop them falling asleep during feeds, or timed naps, really doesn't make any difference other than to cause difficulties when it isn't working. Some parents have even reported mental health issues caused by trying to get babies into routines. Overwhelmingly, the parents I meet say that once they stop fighting against what's happening and learn how to parent in a responsive way (and, importantly, how to cope with that), things become *so* much easier!

If you want to do something to try to support their day/night rhythm emerging, the best thing you can do is ensure lots of daylight during daytime. The circadian rhythm can start to emerge from around Weeks 6 to 8. Most babies will still need lots of feeds overnight, but you may start to notice a bit more of a pattern of night and day around this time.

Feeding responsively, whenever the baby asks and for whatever reason, will usually be sporadic for quite some time, with no predictable routine. But as the weeks go by, you may start to notice a little bit of a pattern emerging perhaps around Week 8 to 10 (but maybe not, so don't worry if you don't). If you want to, you can then start to sculpt that pattern a little to fit your life. For example, you might notice that they're cluster feeding a lot in the evening, but crashing out for a longer sleep once that's done around 10pm perhaps. So you might decide to start a bedtime pattern about 9.30pm, when they have a fresh nappy and clean PJs. Sing them a song, and back on to the boob for a final feed before bed. But if it doesn't flow, or if it works some nights and not others, please don't worry! It really does become a lot easier as they get older. There is no rush to get them into a routine: just let it happen as it happens and you'll find it's much easier.

Cookies and oats for milk production

If you spend any time on internet forums, like parenting Facebook groups, you'll see lots of posts where parents are worried about their milk supply. In response, you'll hear people suggesting that they try eating lots of things with oats in, like porridge and flapjacks, or eat lots of special 'lactation cookies', which are made with ingredients said to be supportive of healthy lactation.

Now, I'm not ever going to tell you to turn down a cookie or a flapjack if someone offers one, but please don't expect it to do much for your milk. What makes you make more milk is removing milk. That's it. No amount of oats or cookies is going to make any difference. So, if you really have problems with low milk supply (and do you, definitely?), you need to try to figure out how to remove more milk (e.g. changing the baby's latch so it's more effective or efficient, or hiring a hospital grade pump). See p. 97 for more.

Infrequent pooing

It's incredibly common to hear people say that breastfed babies don't poo much, and often they say it's because there isn't much waste. But, actually, this isn't true, and causes a lot of difficulty for parents who may be getting mixed messages or incorrect advice. Problems then develop or magnify because the appropriate support hasn't been given and problems have been missed.

From six weeks of age onward, babies *may* develop their own individual stooling pattern within a range of normal. Some babies still go several times a day, some will not go for several days or even longer, and this may still be normal, *if* all else is well.

In the first six weeks, though, we expect them to poo at least twice in 24 hours, though the average number is four. The most common cause of infrequent poo in those early weeks is that they need more milk. If plenty of milk is going in, plenty of poo will be coming out. That's why those of us supporting breast-feeding ask about poo so much, as it's a really good indicator of what's going on!

If pooing is infrequent in those early days or weeks, it's what we call a 'red flag', meaning something that highlights the need for extra investigation. It definitely shouldn't be dismissed as normal without someone trained in breastfeeding assessments watching a full feed to assess milk intake and asking relevant questions about feeding. And please remember that this isn't to criticise you or judge you in any way, it's to support you in making sure feeding is going as well it should.

Sadly, I've worked with so many parents who have been told it's normal for their baby not to poo, only to then find that actually there had been feeding or milk intake problems that could have been sorted much sooner if they hadn't been falsely reassured. If you're in a situation now where your baby isn't pooing as expected in those early weeks, and you've been told it's normal, I would suggest reaching out for trained support. This may be the infant feeding team via your NHS Trust, the National Breastfeeding Helpline, a breastfeeding counsellor or IBCLC lactation consultant – voluntarily or privately. It may well be something very simple that just needs adjusting, so please don't worry, but it's not something that should be ignored. You've chosen to breastfeed, which is awesome, and we want you to be able to continue feeding your baby until you choose to stop, not because things don't go well. Troubleshooting in the early days is a really good way of ensuring things go well in the long term and to get you to your goals.

If you're reading this past the six-week mark, but thinking your baby didn't poo frequently back then, then, again, please don't worry. If you're happy things are going well and your baby is thriving, things might well have rectified themselves naturally. If you're not sure if things are going well, then get yourself a feeding assessment with someone for reassurance.

What you eat causes wind

As we covered in detail elsewhere, milk is made from your blood, not your stomach contents. So, if you eat lots of cabbage, or drink a fizzy drink, *you* might get windy because of the digestion that goes on in your gut, but your baby won't get windy, because they're not having to break down the food and drink – you've done that for them!

What you're eating and drinking gets processed by your body and goes into your blood. Your milk then gets made from your blood. So there's no reason to avoid 'windy' foods, or spicy foods, or any foods at all! Unless, of course, you notice a pattern that when you eat a particular food your baby struggles in the following day or two. If so, see p. 190 for more info.

Babies are lazy feeders

Sometimes babies get labelled as lazy feeders. This might be if they won't latch, if they fall asleep quickly into a feed, or if feeds take a long time. However, all of these things are actually a sign of a feeding problem and not a personality trait!

If your baby won't latch, they're not lazy – it may be that they need to be held in a different way that allows them to open wide enough or at the right angle; they might have a tongue tie, or something else. If they're falling asleep quickly into the feed, it's not because they're lazy, it's because the flow of milk isn't driving them to actively feed. It may be that their latch needs adjusting, or that you need to boost your milk supply for example. And if feeds are taking a long time, it's not because they're lazy – it's because there's a difficulty with how they're accessing the milk, or with milk supply.

If a professional tells you your baby is 'lazy', I'd suggest working with someone else that understands feeding a bit better. Go right back to basics with positioning and latch as per p. 42 and do lots of skin to skin to help.

No such thing as tongue tie

There are still people who don't believe tongue tie exists. I suspect these people haven't ever spoken to someone that has suffered through the difficulties that having a tie can present! Please know that it is a myth that tongue tie doesn't exist and see chapter 12 for more.

Breastfeeding makes your boobs sag

Yep, this one is also a myth! It is pregnancy that causes breast changes, not breastfeeding. Please don't let the future potential appearance of your breasts put you off breastfeeding, as it won't make any difference.

You can't drink alcohol if you breastfeed

You can! For those of you who like an occasional drink, you'll be pleased to know that you can still have a drink or two while you're breastfeeding. Alcohol does pass into breastmilk, but in very very small amounts. A lot of the official guidance suggests that you have the drink as you feed, or just after, so that your body has time to process the alcohol before you feed again. Some experts feel, though, that there is no need to do this, and that actually you could drink a lot more than a few drinks without your milk being detrimental to your baby. However, it's not good for any of us to drink several alcoholic drinks in one go and then try to parent a baby, so it's best avoided.

Do you need to pump your milk and chuck it out ('pump and dump') if you've been drinking? Nope. Partly because the amounts of alcohol that go into the milk are so small, but mainly because alcohol disappears from your milk the same way it does from your blood. You don't need to remove your blood to get rid of the alcohol, and in the same way you don't need to remove your milk. Your body will process it. Cheers!

However, there is one thing that's important to remember: **if you have even one drink, you <u>must not</u> bed-share with your baby**.

Breastfeeding hurts

Well, yep! Breastfeeding can hurt, and it's not uncommon – but that's not because pain is normal. It's not something to expect or something to put up with.

Over the years, when support has been so poor, the message that feeding hurts has been so deeply ingrained into us that we just expect it now. But it really shouldn't. The reason pain is common is that it's tricky to get babies latched; it's a learned skill, that's natural but certainly isn't easy. And if the baby isn't latched properly – it hurts!

If you were able to get a textbook latch 100 per cent of the time, you may have slight discomfort at the start of the feed, but that would be it. However, it's unrealistic to suggest it's going to be perfect every time. It's going to take a bit of time to get right. So, yes, there might be some pain on occasion for some people. However, it's not something to just push through; it's a sign that something isn't right. Listen to your body and get some support.

Breastfeeding makes babies clingy

Our society is so mixed up about babies. There seems to be this thought that they should be made to be as independent as possible as fast as possible. So, if we're breastfeeding, and then our babies want to stay close to us, people often think they're 'clingy' and that it's because they're breastfed. But it's completely natural for our babies to want to stay close to us, and to need us. It's not a sign of a problem.

It's not that breastfeeding makes them clingy. In fact, all evidence suggests quite the opposite! By building a secure attachment, and meeting their needs in a timely and responsive fashion, you're actually going to help them become more independent and confident as they grow up.

Breastfeeding means you can't take medication

Over the years many parents have been told they have to stop breastfeeding (or 'pump and dump') in order to take medications. But, thankfully, in general this isn't true.

Yes, there are certain medications, such as chemotherapy, that are absolutely incompatible with breastfeeding. But, on the whole, a lot of medications are fine, and if there's any question on their safety, there is usually something else that can be used instead. In the UK, we are lucky enough to have the Breastfeeding Network Drugs in Breastmilk service, which has provided multiple factsheets on various medications and conditions. They also have a service to contact specialist pharmacists to discuss what's known about certain medications and breastfeeding, and what alternatives are available. This is open to both parents and health professionals. So, if you need any medication and have concerns about the compatibility with breastfeeding, please know in almost all cases it's possible to continue. If you're told you need to stop, seek a second opinion.

You can't use formula if you breastfeed

Okay, there isn't a straightforward yes or no regarding this one. But it certainly isn't as clear cut as you definitely can't. Lots of parents *do* use formula as part of their feeding journey, very successfully.

Unfortunately, lots of parents also use formula and find it damages breastfeeding and they end up having to move to formula feeding more than they had planned.

Problems that can happen are:

- Bottle preference, meaning your baby refuses the breast but feeds easily and happily from a bottle.

- Feeding difficulties at the breast, because of the different action of feeding from breast and bottle. Babies may experience frustration at differing flow, or you may find you have nipple pain due to adjusted latch.

- 'Top up trap': this is when someone gives some formula, their breasts then get less stimulation and so produce less milk, so they give more formula, and the cycle continues. This can cause breastfeeding to become less and less, and formula feeding to increase.

- Taking a large amount of milk from the bottle and then not being satisfied by a smaller amount at the breast (breastfed babies tend to take little and often).

I'm not saying any of these things to scare you, or put you off if it's what you want to do. But I also don't want you to be unaware and find you have difficulties that you then regret.

Key things to remember if you want or need to use some formula, are:

- If you can, offer the formula after a breastfeed, and even put them back to the breast after the bottle for comfort and relaxation.

- Pace-feed the bottle. See p. 148 for information on this.

- Use the slowest flow teat that's available.

- Keep amounts to a minimum. Be sure to only offer 30–45ml (1–1½ ounces) per hour since they've fed, e.g. if the last feed was two hours ago, offer 60–90ml (2–3 ounces). Try not to offer more than 4 ounces, though, as this can stretch their tummy and make them uncomfortable.

If you want to use formula as part of feeding your baby, of course you can! Many families do.

What I don't want, though, is for you to feel you *have* to use it if you don't want to or hadn't planned to. If that's you, please do get some support with working out other options.

Breastfeeding should come naturally

Breastfeeding is natural, yep. But it's also something that has to be learned. We've said this before, but it bears repeating: breast-feeding is natural like walking, not natural like breathing. So, you need to give yourself time and space to get to grips with it. It's also important to have realistic expectations around breastfeeding, mainly for your own mental health. And by realistic I don't mean that you may not be able to do it; I mean you probably can, but it may take time. It can be weeks or more before you feel like you know what you're doing, and that's okay!

You shouldn't breastfeed when you're ill

This makes sense when you first think about it, so I can understand why this myth is out there. Viruses are contagious, and we try to keep away from others when we have them, and of course we know that babies are precious new little people that we want to protect. But it's actually really important to keep breastfeeding when you're poorly.

Partly this is because avoiding breastfeeding for that time may mean your milk supply decreases. Partly, it's because whatever bug you have, your little one has likely already been exposed to it, so keeping your distance would be a bit pointless anyway. But mainly, it's because your body is so fantastically clever, and the antibodies that you're making in order to fight any infection you've got will be quickly zoomed into your breastmilk to help protect your baby. This means that your baby will either avoid what you've got, or it will be less severe. Isn't that the coolest?

So definitely keep feeding when you're ill. (Though, gosh, I know it's tough!)

Breastfeeding makes it hard for partners to bond

'But how will they bond if they can't feed the baby?' This gets said a lot, but there are *so* many ways to bond with a baby without feeding them. Cuddling, baths together, skin to skin, wearing in a sling, play, singing, going for walks, baby groups, reading books, massage, dancing, talking, telling stories . . . and so much more. They can even cuddle the baby while you feed them if they really want to be involved in feeding time. It's just not true that partners won't bond without feeding, so if you haven't planned giving bottles as part of your journey, please don't feel you have to do it for this reason.

Breastfed babies wake more at night

Nope. Not true at all. In fact, the research shows that if you breastfeed you get *more* sleep on average. Probably because, in the long run, it's quicker and easier to breastfeed at night – you won't have to get up and boil kettles and sterilise equipment. More just 'roll over and pop a boob out and go back to sleep'!

Another reason is that breastmilk contains a hormone that helps babies sleep, and breastfeeding helps you to release a hormone that helps you get back to sleep more quickly too. So, all in all, though it may not feel like it at times, you're not getting less sleep than your friends who formula feed.

Breastmilk is lacking in iron

Iron is vital for normal growth and development. It's one of the micronutrients people are most familiar with, so it's also one of the things we hear talked about with breastmilk and breastfeeding. But the message has got a bit muddled.

The reason for the confusion comes from various places. Firstly, the amount of iron in breastmilk is really small, so it may be understandable to assume that it's not going to be enough. But, when a healthy term baby is born, they have stores of iron that have developed during their time in the womb. These stores start to naturally and slowly deplete from around four to six months of age. Research has been a bit conflicting about this, and for that reason sometimes iron supplements are recommended for breastfed babies from four months. The World Health Organisation, who are considered by most as the leading authority on public health, state there is no need for this, as a general measure; that, as babies start to take iron-rich foods from six months, this will offset the slow depletion of their natural stores.

Another reason iron levels are small is because there are factors in breastmilk (lactoferrin) that actually help the baby to absorb the iron that's available. This is *so* important. Why? Because iron that's left sitting in the gut is delicious food for bacteria, and that leaves the baby susceptible to a variety of infections.

So the short version is that iron is found in small amounts in breastmilk for a reason. It's not meant to be available in huge quantities, because that would be a negative thing.

Another reason for confusion and mixed messages is one that makes me a little . . . exasperated! You see, in the past, and very likely the future too, sadly, the myth around iron not being sufficient in breastmilk has been preyed upon by formula companies (Sidenote: I am not against using formula in the slightest, but I am against the unethical and damaging marketing of the multi-billion pound formula industry). So, we have families hearing (incorrect) messages that their milk isn't providing enough iron for their baby, then an advert comes on showing what huge amounts of iron formula has in it (which, by the way, it needs to have, because it doesn't have the special factors in breastmilk that help absorb it!). Mum then starts to consider if the formula would be better for her baby than her breastmilk . . .

That's why many think it's unethical, because it's not true, and it's making families question their choices unnecessarily. It's not fair. And this is the tip of the iceberg, in honesty; the issues sur-rounding formula marketing are fairly complex. The overriding message to get across is that for the majority of families with a healthy, full-term baby that is growing well, insufficient iron in breastmilk is not something to worry about.

You can't breastfeed if your boobs are too big – or small

The size of your breasts almost always has no correlation with whether you can breastfeed. If you're in the itty bitty titty committee (like me!), you've probably found yourself questioning how on earth your breasts could ever make enough to grow a human. But be assured: small boobs have no less milk-making tissue than bigger ones.

And if your boobs are really big, you might worry about how you're going to be able to get in a comfy position for feeds, or that you might smother the baby, but, honestly, with time, patience and practice, you'll be able to figure out a good way for you. I promise.

> *Top tip:* some people roll up a muslin cloth and put it under their breast to lift it and for added support.

You can't breastfeed if your nipples are inverted or flat

Sometimes it can be more tricky to get breastfeeding started if your nipples are flat or inverted, but for most it's certainly possible. Of course, most of the pictures and videos about latching a baby feature very protruding nipples, which really doesn't help if yours don't look that way!

Some nipples don't have any part that protrudes, so are known as flat, some pull inward toward the breast, and these are known as inverted. And because breastfeeding involves getting the breast really far back into the baby's mouth to trigger the sucking reflex (and keep the breast soft and comfortable), it's easy to imagine it will be harder to do this if the nipple doesn't protrude. But it's not impossible. Some babies have no problems at all feeding from a flat or inverted nipple, and sometimes it's actually a positive thing – it encourages them to latch deeply onto the breast rather than just hanging on the end of the nipple!

You and your baby will need lots of skin-to-skin time, however, to learn about each other's bodies and how they fit best together. Some breast shaping may be needed to assist with latching for some of you too. And, for a few, nipple shields may be a good option, to help give some additional length. However, these should only be used after the baby has had lots of opportunity to try without. See p. 79 for more information on shields.

Breastfeeding is a contraceptive

So, actually, breastfeeding *can* be used as a contraceptive, but *only if* the following conditions are met:

– Baby is under six months old

– Periods haven't returned

– You're feeding responsively and exclusively day and night, i.e. on demand, with no bottles or dummies.

It's also important that you stay close to your baby too. If these conditions are met, then, actually, breastfeeding has been found to be 98 per cent effective as contraception, which is a better percentage than with condoms (though, of course, breastfeeding can't protect from STIs) – it's called the Lactation Amenorhhea Method (LAM).

But, and this is the important bit, as Western parents we often don't meet the conditions for responsive feeding and closeness to our babies, even though we think we might. So there have been many many occasions where pregnancy has happened unplanned because the parents were relying on breastfeeding when perhaps they shouldn't. So, if there is any doubt in your mind whether the conditions are being met, and you don't want a pregnancy, *don't* rely on breastfeeding as a contraceptive.

Pumping tests your supply

What you can pump tells you just one thing – what you can pump. It doesn't tell you what your supply is at all. And, actually, it just tells you what you can pump on that day at that time with that pump . . . as we've seen, not all pumps are created equal, and not all flanges are the right fit!

Babies, on the whole, are much more effective at removing milk from the breast than a pump. This is for a few reasons: one is that the baby's mouth moves in a much more complex way than a pump sucks. But, also, hormones tend to gush much more for a baby, which allows milk to flow, than they will for a pump. Very few people look at their pump and go 'ahhh, it's so cute, I love it so much' the way they do for a baby! Some people can barely pump anything but have babies that are growing beautifully! Pumping *really* isn't a good test of supply.

Conclusion

Honestly, I've barely scratched the surface of the myths that are out there, but these are some that I come into contact with day in, day out, so I felt they would be useful to cover. Essentially, if you hear something about breastfeeding that doesn't seem right to you, question it. It may be nonsense!

Zoe's story

Breastfeeding with my first baby had gone well, so I was quite relaxed about feeding while pregnant with my second child. She was born five days early and it was a lovely birth, with no tearing or anything, so we returned home from hospital quickly and I felt confident that I knew what I was doing feeding-wise. To begin with, she seemed to latch on okay but was fussy, squirmy and didn't seem satisfied.

When she was weighed, she had dropped a bit, but the midwives were happy that this was normal, so we carried on. At three weeks in, she was gaining weight but really slowly and she'd found her thumb. We then entered into a really confusing time of trying to feed, the baby not settling at the breast and then sucking her thumb. This soothed her in the short term but obviously meant she wasn't getting much milk. To be honest, I still don't know what the issue was and, as my husband and I grew more tired and worried, it seemed more difficult to see things clearly. She also seemed far more settled and happy when in my husband's arms. It's fairly obvious in hindsight that this was because he was more relaxed, but at the time it felt like she didn't like me. The advice I was given was to wait between feeds to make sure she was hungry and not feeding for comfort. I now know how much is wrong with that advice, but we dutifully tried to wait, then felt guilty for 'giving in' and feeding. She put on enough weight to not be of any concern to the health visitors, but several times they advised me to give her some formula. I felt increasingly that was my only option, with relatives, friends and health professionals all suggesting that it would solve both our problems. My mother-in-law in particular seemed almost cross with me for not taking this obvious way out. I had my successful feeding experience with my firstborn under my belt, however, and felt genuinely that if I could just work out which tweaks to make we could make it work. So many people had commented on what a 'natural mum' I was with my first, and this difficult situation didn't seem to fit. Surely a 'natural mum' would instinctively know what her baby needed? With the benefit of hindsight, it's clear what tweaks we should have made. If I'd had Lucy around, I'm sure she would have said to offer the breast as often as the baby needed and maybe this simple change would have turned things around for us. It certainly would have made me more relaxed, less guilt ridden, and perhaps the baby would have been more relaxed at the breast as a result. Interestingly, she has since been diagnosed with autism and is very, very particular about food. She also doesn't really like cuddles or physical touch. I do wonder whether that made breastfeeding more of a challenge, but there was no way of knowing at the time. In the end, we fed until exactly 24 weeks (six months), struggling on, feeling like we didn't ever get into a rhythm with it. At six months I breathed a sigh of relief that I'd made it, her daddy started giving her bottles and, frustratingly, she did settle. Out of my three children, her feeding journey was the most challenging, but I'm really glad I persevered for that time. Sometimes we don't really understand what has really happened until much later, I guess.

14

Mental health, birth trauma and when things don't work out as planned

It's no secret that your mental health can be affected when you've had a baby. Lack of sleep, hormones, and societal expectations all play a huge role. It was previously estimated that 1 in 10 of us would be affected by mental health struggles postnatally, but, since the Covid-19 pandemic, the figures are much higher, and are now estimated to be at least 1 in 5.

I'm not a mental health practitioner, but I feel very passionately about this subject, as a sufferer three times over with postnatal anxiety and depression. But I got better, and you can too. And it's completely possible to continue breastfeeding alongside mental health difficulties.

I know this chapter could be a hard read, but please do read it if you can.

Baby blues

This makes it sound so cutesy, but it's really not! A few days after your baby is born, often around the time your milk 'comes in', a lot of us suffer a bit of an emotional crash. Perhaps it's to do with the initial adrenaline and excitement of their arrival calming down. Perhaps it's the hormonal changes of milk production.

Perhaps it's lack of sleep kicking in. Perhaps all of those things or none of them. Whatever it is, it can be tough.

I remember sitting on the sofa feeding my first baby around about Day 4. Her dad had gone to the shop or somewhere similar. The remote control and my drink were out of my reach, and I started to howl and I couldn't stop. At that moment I decided I was the worst mother in the entire *world* because I couldn't even manage to get myself a drink. Seems ridiculous and a bit funny now, but at the time it felt *so* real.

And that's what baby blues can be like: tearful, low, vulnerable feelings, mood swings, snappiness perhaps. Theoretically, these feelings should only last a day, or a few days at most. If it goes on longer than that, then it's something you need to reach out for support with (or before then, if you're worried).

Trying to get as much rest as you can is always helpful (yes, I know that's easier said than done), and eating and drinking plenty is really important too. A lot of us have heard the term 'hangry', for people who get angry when they're hungry, but actually it can cause all manner of negative feelings, so it definitely won't help if you're not eating. Your body needs lots of food and fluids at this time, because not only are you healing from birth, but also working on making lots of milk, and may not be getting as much sleep as you need. Try to eat little and often; have people make food for you and/or have some snack bars dotted around the place to grab. Some parents find having large bottles of water in several places in every room helpful too. But it's important to make sure those around you know this may happen, and how to help you if it does. Oh, and have the remote control handy ;)

Puerperal psychosis

I just want to touch on this briefly, so that you, or those around you, are aware of the signs. It's a scary topic to discuss, but I think every parent that has ever had this illness wishes it was discussed more so that other parents, and their own support network, would know what to look out for.

Puerperal psychosis (PP) is a mental health condition that can happen in the first few days or weeks after you've had your baby. PP is severe, and an emergency situation, and will be treated in hospital, or a psychiatric hospital setting. It differs from baby blues or depression mainly because of its severity, but also includes the symptom of either delusions, hallucinations, or mania. Delusions are the belief that things are real that are not – for example, being convinced you're the King. Hallucinations are having visions or hearing voices that are not there. Mania is a type of hyperactivity that feels inappropriate for the situation, and often involves being out of touch with reality. For example, deciding that 3am is the perfect time to start sorting out the kitchen cupboards.

This illness can happen to *anyone*, and can be very sudden in its onset (but not always). The parent suffering is often not aware they are unwell. And while it can happen to anyone, we know that those with existing bipolar disorder have a higher rate. The Action on Postpartum Psychosis website is full of information, including common early signs, and is well worth a look.

Anxiety

Having a new baby can be a very anxious time. There's lots to learn in a short time-frame, and stuff that's usually really important to us! There are so many different ways to do things, views on what you should and shouldn't do, pressure to do X, Y and Z, and, at the centre of everything, this precious little person that we want to do our very best for; it's only natural that we'll feel anxious from time to time.

For some parents, though, it can become more than that and they may suffer with anxiety, an actual mental health condition, where those worries become disproportionate and out of control. Perhaps worries about health, food, or not wanting to leave the house because it doesn't feel safe, for example. It may not be related to the baby or parenting, but it might. It may be that those around you notice your struggles before you do, so do try to hear what your loved ones are trying to say if they tell you that they're concerned about you.

Those with babies under one year old will be prioritised for mental health support, such as talking therapies. There are also medications that are compatible with breastfeeding, if you and your doctor felt this was the best thing for you. I know how difficult it can be reaching out, but I promise you it will be worth it.

Depression

Similar to the reasons for anxiety, there can be days when having a baby can make you feel low. But if this is happening often, increasingly, and/or you're struggling to enjoy things that you normally would, please do reach out.

Often friends, family, and even health professionals may suggest stopping breastfeeding to help you feel better. It's said with best intentions and kindness at heart, but we know that stopping breastfeeding won't help make things better for the vast majority of people, and can actually make things worse.

We know that parents who don't reach their own breastfeeding goals have higher rates of postnatal depression, and often report feelings of grief and loss.

There are *absolutely* ways to continue breastfeeding while suffering with depression. That's not to suggest it's easy, and I wish I could change that for you, I really do. But I can promise that getting through this hard patch will be worth it and is definitely possible, even though it may not feel that way. Do, however, try to communicate with your friends and family, and get them to help as much as you can.

Postnatal OCD

You may have heard of obsessive compulsive disorder (OCD). The condition is often assumed to be to do with an obsession with cleanliness and needing to repeatedly wash hands. For some people it can be that, of course, but actually OCD can present in lots of different ways. Having obsessive thoughts – negative ones – and needing to carry out certain compulsions can affect up to 2 per cent of us postnatally. That's 2 in every 100: much higher than might be expected.

It might be that you're affected in a way unrelated to the baby, such as needing to turn a light switch on and off a certain number of times, or it may be related to the baby, like feeling you need to check very frequently that they are breathing, for example. So, if you notice you're having negative thoughts, and that you're having to act on them with certain behaviours to 'cancel them out', it may be that you're suffering with postnatal OCD. It can be very debilitating and difficult, but can be supported. As ever, it's important to reach out, and to do so as early as possible, if you feel something is going on for you

Intrusive thoughts

Have you ever been standing somewhere high up and thought 'I could jump off this'? Or walking along a pavement with a friend and thought 'I could push them into the road'? Scary, horrible thoughts, right?! But no intention of actually acting on them. An extraordinarily high percentage of people get these. They're called 'intrusive thoughts' and they're really common. And they can happen more often at times when you're stressed, tired and hormonal . . . so when you've just had a baby is a prime opportunity, for sure!

Intrusive thoughts can be really unpleasant, and because of this we often keep them to ourselves. I mean, when you're trying to make polite conversation about baby massage class, you don't usually drop in 'I often think about throwing my baby down the stairs', do you? So we keep these thoughts to ourselves, and then none of us realise how often others suffer with these thoughts too, but, honestly, you're *not* alone.

Usually, the thoughts centre around hurting the baby, accidentally or on purpose, but they can also take on a sexual nature too, like worrying we might touch the baby inappropriately during a nappy change, which can be really distressing for parents. The key here is that you have no intention of acting on these thoughts, and that they're awful or disgusting to you. In that sense, the thoughts are no danger to anyone, they're just thoughts. Horrible thoughts, but just thoughts.

The time when they can be more of a problem is if you feel that you may actually act on them, if they're so distressing to you that they're affecting your mental health, or if you're having to carry out certain behaviours to make them go away. If this sounds familiar to you, please speak to someone for some help.

Will they take my baby away?

No. It's understandable that you may worry about this, because there has been a lot of stigma around mental health and parenthood for a long time. But it just doesn't happen. It doesn't.

Even in cases of the most severe, life changing and debilitating mental health struggles, absolutely every effort is made to keep parents and babies together. Thousands and thousands of parents every week are supported with mental illness, and you can be too.

Birth trauma and the effect on breastfeeding

Birth can be difficult sometimes, and I think we're all aware of that. Occasionally, though, it can be a traumatic experience that affects us mentally, both short- and long-term. It can present itself a little like PTSD, affecting our mood, ability to cope, and involve having flashbacks, difficulty sleeping, feeling anxious and 'jumpy', and more.

I suffered my own birth trauma with my third baby. I had been a midwife for many years, and been through a lot of difficult and even life-threatening births. But my own experiences changed me for ever. So I just want to say: if you're going through this, I'm so sorry – I know how hard it is.

Inevitably, it's possible for breastfeeding to be impacted in these situations. Physical barriers, such as separation at birth, being too unwell to feed, or NICU stays, for example, can have an impact on getting feeding established. There is a huge list of physical barriers to breastfeeding that are related to birth trauma, and parents will likely need extra support, even with the basics.

The mental barriers to breastfeeding should not be under-estimated either. You may have lost faith in your body, in its abilities. You may also have lost faith in the system that is meant to support you. You may feel like you're the one that needs mothering, but instead you have to try to put your mental energy into breastfeeding, which is, even at the best of times, really hard and intense at first.

For some parents, they feel it's not the right choice for them to breastfeed now, because they simply cannot face another trauma if things don't go well. And, as health professionals, we absolutely understand and respect those decisions.

Ideally, someone will have been able to have a gentle discussion with the traumatised parent, so that the individual concerned can be sure their decision is a truly informed choice. As we've seen, there are many parents that regret not breastfeeding, or stopping too soon, so this discussion is useful if parents are happy to talk it through. For parents that have undergone birth trauma, it may be that they'd be happy to carry on doing some expressing for a little while, in a manageable way, so as to keep the door open for breastfeeding further down the line, if they wish to. It doesn't have to be all or nothing.

For a lot of parents, it can work the other way too: the need to breastfeed becomes even more important to them. They need to be able to trust in their body again; need to give their baby the best they can; need to reclaim ownership of the journey into parenthood. The drive within them can become overwhelming and can be used to overcome the challenges that can be faced, and maybe even draw strength from within that they didn't know they had.

Sometimes, though, the trauma can manifest itself in a focus on breastfeeding. There can even be elements of obsession surrounding milk intake, weights, timings of feeds for example. On the surface, feeding may be going well, but when you discuss it further, it becomes apparent that they're having a hard time.

Communicating with your partner, your family, and your friends is going to be so important after birth trauma. You need looking after, so let them look after you, let them know what you need (if you know). Make sure that your midwife, health visitor or GP are aware as well, in case things don't improve. Request a referral to the mental health support team for talking therapies – a lot of NHS Trusts have a 'birth afterthoughts'-type of debriefing service, which can be really beneficial. And get a referral to the infant feeding team too, as breastfeeding difficulties, as we know, are best sorted early on.

When breastfeeding doesn't go as planned

If you're reading this because this is you, I'm really sorry. It can hurt a lot, and people don't always seem to understand.

Unfortunately, in the Western world, we have very poor breast-feeding support on the whole, and for a lot of parents breastfeed-ing doesn't go the way they had hoped, and ends before they had wanted. In fact, the last big survey that was done found that 80 per cent of those that stopped breastfeeding said they did so before they had planned to.

Our breastfeeding rates in the UK are very low, with only 1 per cent estimated to still be exclusively breastfeeding at six months. And that's not because we don't want to be breastfeeding, it's because something has caused us to stop. But it is *not* your fault. Do not think this for even one second – it's not.

I can assure you that it's not because you didn't try hard enough. It is not because you're not strong enough. It is not because you're not a good parent. It is because you were in a system that is broken, and not able to appropriately support you to reach your goal. And I'm sorry – it's not okay that it's like this.

Parents often describe that they get grief-like feelings when breastfeeding hasn't gone well or has stopped before they were ready. Others explain that it was actually a traumatic experience for them. You might find yourself trying to ignore or minimise these feelings, perhaps because you feel like you shouldn't be experiencing them. But please let yourself grieve for your loss. Let yourself process the trauma you've gone through. It's important to feel these feelings and process them properly.

Friends, family and even health professionals often try to make you feel better by saying things that actually may not help. For example, remarking on how well you did to get to X amount of days, or Y amount of weeks, which, while said with the best intention and, arguably, very true, completely fails to recognise that you may be very aware of how well you've done but that wasn't what you wanted. You wanted to *choose* to stop feeding, not feel like you had no choice because of pain, or milk supply issues, for example.

They may also say that formula is fine to use and not to worry about breastfeeding anyway. Of course, formula *is* fine, but again, it wasn't what you wanted. In trying to be helpful, often our thoughts and feelings are minimised or pushed aside.

I would strongly suggest speaking with someone if you're struggling. Breastfeeding counsellors, and IBCLCs, can help with debrief sessions. This is where they listen to your experiences, help you unpick what happened and why, and, very importantly – validate what you're feeling. It's a safe space for you to explore what you're feeling, judgement free. Parents have found that even a one-off session has helped them move forward, so please do explore this if you're struggling. Some NHS Trusts also offer a debrief service, or your health visitor may be able to provide listening visits too. And Dr Amy Brown has written a book about breastfeeding grief, called *Why Breastfeeding Grief and Trauma Matter*, if you would like further reading.

Relactation

It can be a difficult topic to discuss at this point, but I want to touch on relactation here, just in case it helps someone. For a lot of you it may be that you've moved away from breastfeeding, and while it may not be what you wanted, you might be comfortable with that now, or you may want to avoid going back to breastfeeding for fear of further difficulties or upset. For others, they would like to try breastfeeding again, but often aren't aware that it's possible, which is why I mention it here.

In a lot of circumstances it is possible to relactate, which means to get milk supply up and running again and breastfeed the baby. It doesn't matter how long ago you stopped, as you should still be able to produce milk again. Though I won't minimise the fact that it can take a lot of work and determination.

If you're considering relactation, I'd strongly advise you get some support on how to move forward. The key things to consider will be:

- Getting baby to latch

- Getting milk supply boosted

Have a look at the chapters on latching and expressing for support with this, and the book *Relactation* by Lucy Ruddle may also be helpful.

Conclusion

If you don't feel quite like yourself and it's concerning you, please know that it's not your fault, and it can get better. One of my biggest hopes for this book is that even one person feels empowered to get the help they need. Let it be you. You deserve the support, I promise.

Hannah's story

Postnatal OCD

Initially I was very anxious something was going to happen to my baby, but this soon evolved into compulsive behaviours and horrific and realistic intrusive thoughts. I developed an intense fear of water and a certainty when driving that I'd not put the baby in the car but had left her somewhere on the side of the road. I'd stop the car to check she was there only to convince myself that, upon checking, I'd taken her out of the car and would have to stop again to check minutes later. I knew this wasn't right or normal. Breastfeeding not only gave me something positive to remind me that there was something I was doing right every single day but also calmed my anxiety.

Holding my baby close at the breast gave me a sense we were working this out together and made me feel less lonely and ashamed, because the person who loved me and relied on me most didn't hold any judgement against me. She just wanted me to feed her and so I did. It was the simplest thing to cling to and I'm sure I'd have felt worthless were I unable to continue. It really was the one thing that I knew was good about me as a mother.

15
For partners, friends and family

Partners, friends and family, this chapter is dedicated to you. You are going to make *such* a difference to how breastfeeding and those early days of parenthood go, and you're going to be absolutely fantastic. I know, however, that you might be feeling a lot of things, and have a lot of questions about breastfeeding. So I've put together some bits you might find useful.

How partners might feel

The first thing to know is that whatever you feel is absolutely valid and normal. It might be happiness, fear, confusion, exhaustion . . . probably a mix of a lot of things! You're not expected to know everything, and it's okay to feel a bit lost! You'll be finding your feet and it takes a bit of time. Be patient and kind to yourself while you settle in.

The fact that you're reading this and wanting to understand and know a bit more shows just how wonderful you're going to be, so please try not to worry.

I absolutely believe in you, and that you can help them with what they need, so I've put together this information for you to help. This is what real families tell me that helped them.

We'll also look at how you might feel and what you might experience.

> *'I soon realised it wasn't as easy as we expected it would be, and it made me feel quite powerless. Getting help to sort out the breastfeeding was the best thing we did, I think we would have given up without and regretted it if we did. Secretly, I was glad not to have to mess about with bottles!'* – Andy, dad to Jamie and Charlotte.

> *'I felt amazed and overwhelmed at this new life, but it was such a big responsibility (and I'm not terrifically responsible). It's a bit of a cliché, but it does change everything: your focus, your life, your sleeping patterns, but mostly it's just pretty wonderful. The biggest help with breastfeeding was the local support group.'* – Phil, dad to Emily.

How you can help

Doing chores – It might be that your partner is under the baby feeding a *lot* at first (or even for a longer stretch than you might expect), so there really will be minimal time (and inclination) for them to do much else. Laundry, cleaning, shopping, washing up, hoovering . . . that stuff is going to be the absolute bottom priority and will need someone else to take it over. It really makes a massive difference, so do as much as you can.

Take the mental load – This is a *biggie*. You're going to be doing stuff practically, which is absolutely wonderful, but if your partner or family member is having to organise it all or think about it all, that can actually be almost as tiring as doing it themselves. For example, asking what needs doing immediately means that your partner is the one 'in charge' of everything and you're the helper. Don't be the helper: take it all over, including the organising and thinking ahead. That's not to say they can't be involved, of course they can, just try to think, plan ahead and anticipate what's needed.

Gratitude – I get told this quite often, and it's something so simple that seems to really help. It's saying thank you, or showing your gratitude. 'When he said thank you to me for working so hard to get breastfeeding started, it really helped keep me going' is something I've been told before.

Think about what they might need – you already know your partner is going to be on the sofa or in bed a lot and might not be able to access the things they want or need, so try to think for them. Could you fill up drinks bottles, bring snacks? Might a stretch of the legs be needed – could you offer to hold the baby? Think ahead to what might be needed or helpful. And if you don't know, ask! A very simple 'what can I do to help?' can make a world of difference.

Get up during the night feeds – This was really key for a lot of parents, who told me they really appreciated it when their partner got up with them during night feeds. For company, for moral support, to help get drinks, cushions, snacks etc.

Empower them – It's very likely there will be times when the words 'I can't do it, it's too hard' or something similar will be uttered. Getting breastfeeding established can be really tough and very tiring, so remember your role in empowering your partner/family/friend. Some words of encouragement from you can make all the difference. For example: 'He told me I was the expert in my baby and to follow my instincts.'

Get a doula – A postnatal doula is a professional who works with families in a support role in the early weeks and months after a baby arrives. They might help with feeding, housework, shopping, massage, cooking, mental health support and more. They're a bit like an incredibly helpful and knowledgeable auntie. They are a paid support service, so this is not viable for everyone, but they often have different support packages available, from coming in for a couple of hours once a week to coming in for a few hours every day. Doula UK is a great place to look for someone in your area.

Order meal kits – There's lots of these great meal kit services available now, either with pre-portioned ingredients with recipes that arrive ready to be quickly put together, or deliveries of home-style cooked foods that just need reheating. A lot of families tell me that they really appreciate these in the early weeks post birth.

Look after the animals – Got a dog? Do the walks. Got cats? Feed them. Got horses? Go and do . . . whatever horses need! Take over the animal care and it will be highly valued.

Get familiar with the sling or carrier – Okay, so you can't feed the baby, but you can definitely hold the baby close and provide comfort, which is an enormous amount of what the fourth trimester is about. Babies want to be held close 24/7 at first, and you can do a big chunk of that. What helps hugely is having a comfy sling or carrier.

Babies that are held in slings cry less and grow faster, and parents report better mental health and feel better able to cope. Trust me on this: a sling can be a game changer.

Some areas have sling libraries, where you can try different ones, and even hire or borrow for short or long spells if you don't want to invest, or would like to try before you buy. They can help you with how to get the most comfortable use too, both for you and the baby. And, of course, how to make sure you're using it safely.

> 'I loved *the sling. It took us a little while to find the right one, but once we did it was like a light had been flicked on. To this day I still miss going out at teatime with Toby in the sling for a walk while giving his mum some time in the bath.'*
> – Ian, dad of Toby.

Mum or mother-in-law coming to stay – Well, for some this would be a dream come true, having their mum or mum-in-law come and stay for a week or two. For others it would be a living nightmare! So the most important thing is to *ask*. Would that be something they would like? Have an honest and open conversation about it, and accept their answer without judgement or emotion.

Agree things in advance – A lot of families tell me that having a discussion during pregnancy and getting things agreed in advance can be really supportive once the baby has arrived. Having clear guidelines, boundaries, tasks etc, where everyone knows who is doing what and when, can clear a lot of the mental load.

> 'When *she was still pregnant, we talked about who would do what once we were parents so that it didn't all fall to one person. She knew that ordering the online shop was my thing and not something she needed to think about unless I asked for her help.'*– Chris, dad of Sarah.

Do baby care – Sure, you can't do the feeding, but you can do literally everything else, if needed. Winding, cuddles, nappy changes, bathing, skin to skin, changing clothes, snuggling them at 4am when they get grunty and squirmy and need to be held close and upright!

Prioritise breastfeeding – So many of the parents I've worked with have told me that this is important. They really need their partner and family to understand that breastfeeding is a priority, or perhaps even *the* priority. The early weeks are so very important for getting feeding established, and missing that window can be catastrophic. Breastfeeding very often becomes hugely important once the baby has been born, like a deep instinctive need. It's not just 'I'd like to breastfeed', it's 'I need to breastfeed, I *need* to make this work no matter what'. Understanding that, and being able to prioritise feeding, and supporting feeding, will mean an awful lot.

Be their advocate – Navigating those early weeks with a new baby can be tricky, and because there can be a lot of views, opinions and emotions involved, from everyone around you, it can feel a bit like a minefield. Advocating for them, when they feel they cannot, has been something that was mentioned as really helpful and supportive. For example, if your partner has nipple pain and is told it's normal, they may really value you helping by speaking up to say that you know it's not normal, and where can you get help.

Don't let her quit – Now, when I say this, I don't actually mean that you can 'let' her do anything or not, of course, as the choice is totally hers. What I mean is that, when times get tough, and they will, she might ask for some formula, or say she's going to stop breastfeeding, despite the fact that you know how desperate she was to keep going. So help her get over that bump. Support her, empower her, praise her, let her know that it's going to get better and you're going to do everything in your power to help.

Get her food and drink, and hold the baby so that she can shower and nap. If the baby is cluster feeding, try using a lying-down feeding position and watching over them so that she can sleep while she feeds, knowing you're watching the baby. It's amazing the difference 12–24 hours can make, and she'll thank you for keeping her going.

Learn about what breastfeeding looks like in 2023! – Things are so very different now to when the baby's grandparents had babies (i.e. had you!). There have been drastic changes, in fact. And this can lead to confused messages between your new family and your parents and in-laws. Previously, we were told to only feed every four hours, and let them have only a few minutes on each side. Now we're encouraged to take the baby's lead and let them feed whenever they ask for as long as they want. We do this because we know it's not only beneficial for breastfeeding and milk supply, but also for the baby's brain and emotional health too.

It can be really hard for previous generations not to feel worried, or even upset or offended, at the changes that have happened, as it can feel like a criticism of past methods. But it's simply that we know more now, and so we're going with what we know.

Read up, or investigate what breastfeeding is like now, so that you can fully support what they need and help your partner to navigate conversations with parents and grandparents.

> 'It was very different to when I had my babies, and I found it difficult to understand how things could have changed so much. I must admit I felt very worried at times about the way they were doing things, but I had to trust them to learn to parent their own way.' – Marilyn, grandma to 7.

Ask whether they want solutions, or for you just to listen –
Oof, this is huge. If she's upset, angry, frustrated, struggling in
any way, don't assume she wants answers or solutions. Sometimes
we need to complain how hard it is, how tired we are, how
claustrophobic it is, but that doesn't mean we want to stop. It
might be that, yes, absolutely she wants you to offer suggestions
about how to move forward, but don't assume that. Ask first.

For family members and friends . . .

Avoid giving unsolicited advice – This is the number-one thing
that parents say can actually make them quite upset: offering
advice that they didn't ask for. Suggesting that they give formula,
say, or express milk for a bottle. Suggesting that they sleep train.
Telling them they're holding the baby too much. Giving opinions
on their parenting, or recommending things they should do
because 'we did it, and we're fine'. It's so important that, just as
with the advice for partners above, we ask what they need from
us. Do they *want* our advice?

Don't question how often the baby feeds – The baby is going
to feed a lot. And I really do mean a lot, and overwhelmingly
this is completely normal. When parents are asked 'you're
feeding again?' or told 'he can't be hungry again!', it demoralises
them, makes them worry and question everything, and it isn't
actually true. Breastfeeding is not just about food, but also thirst,
comfort, sleep, security, and so much more. It's a wonderful
parenting tool and we're encouraged to feed whenever they
show cues, or whenever we need to. Trust them that they know
what to do.

If you really are concerned about how often they're feeding,
you could consider signposting the family to someone who

supports infant feeding to work out if all is well for them. For example, a gift voucher for an IBCLC, or find details of their local support group.

Avoid visits, especially unannounced – In those early weeks, there are a lot of people wanting to visit and it can be really overwhelming. You will be the absolute favourite people of the new family if you let them know you're in no rush, and would like to visit at a time that suits them, and for just a short time. Let them know you'll expect to be given things you can do to help while you're there! If they have to cancel at short notice, even though it's so disappointing, try to be understanding, as they probably feel bad for letting you down.

Oh, and if you're at all under the weather, even if it's just a bit of a sniffle or a cold, rearrange your visit unprompted, as they could really do without the added strain of catching a cold at the moment.

Hold the video calls – Covid saw a massive increase in the amount of video calls, of course. Video communication seems to have slipped into our way of life now, but, actually, many new parents are finding it quite stressful. It can feel quite intrusive, especially if unplanned. So try to keep them to a minimum, if you can, and make sure they've been agreed in advance rather than come as a surprise. And remember that your friends or family will probably be in their pyjamas, and that's a good thing!

Wait for updates – It's incredibly exciting having a new baby in the mix, and wanting to know all the news is understandable! Asking for lots of updates on what's happening and how they all are can prove tricky, though. If new parents have got ten people asking, it can be pretty overwhelming, and they need to be concentrating on themselves at the moment. Rest assured that, if they had things they wanted to share, or had the chance to, they would and they will. It doesn't mean you're not important to them, it's just those overwhelming early days!

Don't mention body size or weight – After having a baby, your body looks and feels very different to how it did pre-pregnancy. There's a lot of pressure on parents to try to get their body 'back' and to lose weight and have a flat stomach as soon as possible. It's hugely unhelpful and completely inappropriate, I'm sure you'll agree.

You can help with this, however, by not mentioning postpartum body or weight loss at all. It just doesn't need to come up. Let's focus on how we can support their health and wellness instead.

Don't suggest formula or bottles – When our loved ones are struggling, we'd do anything we can to make it better. The new family are undoubtedly grateful for your support. One thing that they may have asked, though, is that formula isn't suggested as a way of making things easier. It can be really detrimental to getting breastfeeding established, but also, very importantly, it's not what they want to do. There are lots of other ways to help though, as listed above. Please don't assume.

Don't suggest a night off – It may seem a fantastic solution to the exhaustion and difficulty of new parenthood, but offering to take the baby for a night will actually make things more difficult. Keeping them all together is so important for a new family unit.

Don't take the baby – If you're asked to visit, don't take the baby without being offered. We all want a snuggle as soon as we can, but sometimes that means being really patient and possibly not even getting to hold them at all. The whole family are the priority, not cuddles with the newest member.

Know it's okay if they're not happy all the time – There's an enormous pressure on families to be making 'picture perfect' memories with their new baby, but, in reality, it can all be a bit of an exhausted, emotional mess. They're absolutely allowed to struggle, and to complain, and to cry. You just listening will be so wonderful to them.

Be comfortable with breastfeeding – There's gonna be a lot of boob-out time! They may be fine feeding around you, but sometimes they may want to be alone to do it, especially when they're getting started out. If you're unsure what they want you to do, just ask. But, honestly, they'll likely just be focusing on getting the baby fed and not worried about much else.

Don't send flowers – Oh, gosh, I love flowers so much, but, actually, it's not what you need when you've had a baby! If you get loads of bunches, where are you going to put them? Give them a gift voucher for the money instead!

Best gifts

If you want to buy a gift, there are definitely some things that go down better than others. (For me, it was a hamper of the foods I didn't eat during pregnancy!), but here are some other suggestions:

'A massive drink bottle with a straw!'

'An insulated mug to keep my drinks hot'

'Preprepared meals'

'A voucher for a lactation consultant'

'Takeaway vouchers'

'Some visits from a postnatal doula'

'A cleaner!'

'Meal subscription'

'A night light'

Conclusion

So, that's some things that families have shared with me about what's been helpful for them, and hopefully it's got you thinking a bit! Every family is different, though, and what's right for one won't be right for another. And, of course, not all of these will be relevant, but you'd be surprised how much is.

I can't stress enough how important it is to communicate in a calm, honest and loving way, and to accept your loved one's answers, thoughts and feelings without judgement. You are going to be amazing, I have no doubt about it!

Damien's story

'Our oldest, Elijah, was a constant feeder when he was born, which, as you can imagine, was exhausting for my partner Laura. She was, however, determined to breastfeed for as long as possible, so she started by being up almost all night feeding. Again she was ultra-determined to breastfeed, so the first thing we did was to marry up Elijah's bed so that she could just roll over to feed. From my perspective, I also found this tiring, but, after the odd strop, realised I had to just shut up and deal with it! I don't know if feeding had an impact on Elijah's sleeping, but eventually it got unbearable for Laura, so she reluctantly decided to express and store milk in the fridge. This meant she could sleep, as I would get up in the night with Elijah and take him into the lounge and feed him. Obviously this made me extremely tired – not good when I was in medical sales and spent most of my week on the road – but it made me understand the sacrifice Laura was going through. This was our life for the first year with Elijah, but once we got pregnant with Austin, we put Elijah onto formula. To this day, Elijah, at ten years old, still takes an age to fall asleep, but on the plus side I know all the words to *In The Night Garden!*

Ian's story

It's safe to say I was geared up for a full-on 100 per cent breast-fed baby journey. My wife has always been very pro-breastfeeding, and I knew we'd be going for exclusive breastfeeding, from even early in the pregnancy. She'd breastfed her two older children (my stepdaughters) with differing degrees of success, stopping before she was ready first time out (on account of returning to work). I didn't want this to happen again, as I was worried about the effect it could have on her mental health.

I was enthusiastic about bottle feeding with expressed milk, for sure. I had ideas before Toby's birth that I would step up to the plate like the best dad and husband ever, feeding whenever I could so she would be able to get her rest when she needed it.

Things changed after we had a traumatic birth, however. We opted for a home birth and there were complications, which led to us having a stay in special care/NICU for Toby's first week or so of life. During this time I couldn't stay in the hospital with them overnight, so I had to be more of a remote support, rather than the absolute all-hours hands-on support that I'd envisioned myself being. We tried to give a bottle of expressed milk at times, but our son just wouldn't take a bottle – it seemed he was determined to exclusively breastfeed as well! While this didn't really have as much of an impact on the day-to-day as I'd expected

– my wife had really embraced the breastfeeding aspect and was loving it, despite being exhausted – it hit me harder than I thought it would. I really felt like I couldn't help enough, or that I was failing her as a partner at times. Like my son's bottle refusal was my fault, and a burden that I was unnecessarily placing on my wife's shoulders. I know now (and wish I'd known then) that the traumatic birth had really affected my mental health, more than I was willing to admit. That stupid manly attitude of 'just man up' had reared its head, in the wake of depression and PTSD.

The good news was that, once out of the hospital, our baby boy was absolutely thriving being an exclusively breastfed baby. I loved seeing my wife's manner change when the hormones hit her after a minute or so of him being latched on. I loved watching the two of them bond in this way – I knew I'd never have that same connection, but I had such a wonderful connection of my own that I was, for the most part, very secure in what I was doing as a dad. But I kept getting bitten by the old feeling of thinking I wasn't helping enough – every time we had a night wake and I couldn't settle him back down, in the day when he just wanted to be with mummy, or for those first few seconds of my wife *having* to breastfeed, which hit every now and then with a roll of the eyes and a sigh, before that wonderful oxytocin hit came through.

In all honesty, though, were I asked for advice, I'd say there's nothing in your parenting toolkit quite like breastfeeding, as I found out time and again. Sometimes simply nothing else will do, and that's not only normal, it's *okay*, and makes you no less of a dad! Use your rational inner voice and ditch the ego – you're not failing because you aren't able to get a bottle in the little one's mouth. Keep on supporting your wife and kid in whatever way you can, as it all helps.

16

Coming out of the fourth trimester

Here are some of the things I've heard parents coming out of the fourth trimester say:

'The realisation that things had got a load easier without you really noticing.'

'I felt amazing, purely because I knew I'd survived one of the hardest parts.'

'Change was gradual. I expected a sudden change but it was nothing noticeable.'

'I felt emotional and a bit shell shocked. It was really tough for us. It still is.'

'I'm not sure we ever came out of it! She still wants cuddles and feeds 24/7!'

'We started to get some sleep at last.'

'Things didn't get easier even though people said they would.'

'Getting a little myself back again. Just a little.'

'Conflicting feelings. Sadness that the newborn stage was over, but looking forward to moving forward.'

'A blur. Just one long, sleep-deprived blur.'

'I put pressure on myself that I should be able to do more out of the newborn stage, when really I couldn't and that was okay.'

As you head toward the end of the first few months, you'll probably feel like some areas you're nailing it, and others you still have no clue what you're doing. Congratulations on being a very normal parent! You may also find that, just as you feel like you know what you're doing, things change and you feel a bit lost again. I'll give you an example of this.

10–12 weeks

Around 10–12 weeks is a common time for me to get requests for support, because of breast refusal behaviours and fractious feeds among other things. Here's what we often figure out.

Babies discover their hands around this age, and spend a lot of time with them jammed into their mouth. Because this also creates a lot of dribble, it's often mistaken for early teething (some babies really are teething, but for most it's just developmental).

For the entirety of their life up to this point you've known 'hands in the mouth' as a cue to offer a feed, so you put them to the breast and . . . well, a few outcomes tend to happen. Sometimes, they feed. They were hungry. It was the right decision to offer the breast and you feel reassured. Though, equally, what can sometimes happen is they feed . . . but, wow, are they distracted. They keep popping off to have a look about. The world is just too exciting. There's serious FOMO going on.

What can often happen, however, and this is what's really difficult, is they get *mad*. They latch on a bit, but cry and thrash and pull off. They're grumpy, and the boob normally works to calm them, so you keep persisting. But they just get even madder. You're now left utterly confused and upset because your baby is not just refusing to feed, but seemingly hates it.

You may also be worried because your baby has had less milk than usual, so keep offering, but then your baby just gets madder still, and you end up in an anxious tearful spiral. It can be particularly worrying if your baby is having a long stretch of sleep without feeds, which is more common around this age. So, here's what I suggest trying: stop offering.

Yep, I know. It's not often while breastfeeding that we don't live by the mantra of 'if in doubt, whip it out'. But for this age group, temporarily, it can be useful.

That's not to say you should restrict feeds, not at all. If they want feeding, then, of course, feed. It's more about relearning what their cues are now, and recognising that, actually, they often have a reduction in feeds around now and are capable of longer intervals between.

So, when you offer and they get mad, it's very often because they just don't want it at this point. It may be that they're tired, or bored. Previously, feeding would sort these, but at the moment it doesn't. It's usually only temporary. Continuing to offer when they don't want to feed can cause more upset and then end up with breast refusal. They won't starve themselves, I promise; they will take milk when they need it. Sometimes offering while they're sleeping can work, if you're really concerned (sometimes referred to as a 'dream feed'), but mostly their behaviour is being caused by the fact that they're just not newborns any more.

Keep an eye on those nappies, as ever, if it's coming out, then it's going in! And if they've been growing out of their clothes over the last few months, hopefully you are reassured that they're gaining weight well too. But if you feel your baby hasn't been growing, or you're aware of issues with weight gain, it may be a good time to access some well-trained support.

The most important things is to trust your baby and to trust your body.

In my experience, this is usually one of those weird bumps in the breastfeeding journey where the goalposts suddenly seem to move. Be kind to yourself and give yourself some time to get used to this change. Oh, and if this stuff isn't what's happening, that's okay too!

Four-month-olds

Four-month-olds are *glorious*! Full of personality and charm, and busy busy busy. They're developing at a rate of knots as well. And this can sometimes be a bit of a challenge for some families. Not everyone, of course, and babies are very individual. But I think it's worth sharing some thoughts on this age group, in case you're having some difficulties.

So you've got to the 12/13-ish week mark and, just as people had said, things were actually a little brighter for a lot of you. The intense newborn period calms down, and you start to feel a little more confident that you may sort of know what you're doing after all. You're into the swing of things, shall we say? That's not to say it's easy – oh no, no, no! – it's still extremely full on, but often in a more manageable way. You're able to leave the house a little bit more easily, the baby is generally happier and a bit more predictable, and feeding is usually, on the whole, a relaxed experience that you now actually look forward to (if nothing else, so you can sit down and watch Netflix, or scroll through your phone). Best of all, you may even be getting some sleep! Frequent feeds *may* have calmed down a little too. You might be feeling a lot more refreshed than you were, perhaps considering having seven more babies because yours is so fantastic.

Anyway, you potter along like this for a few weeks and then *boom*! It seems like someone swaps your baby for a different one. Let's look at some of the . . . interesting behaviours that show up around this time.

It often feels, at this age, like you can't do anything to please your baby, or if you can, it's not for very long. It's like they're bordering on the edge of grumpy fairly continuously. When you feed them, they don't just snuggle down, glug some milk and fall asleep anymore – they latch on, latch off, look around for a while, cry because they want to latch back on, cry because the milk isn't coming fast enough, or start to pinch and tug at the breast. The milk flows, they pop off to look at the dog, then cry because your milk squirted them in the face. They latch back on, take a bit, pop off and grin at you for a while. You figure they must be finished so put your boob away, they cry, you get it back out, they take three sucks and look at the dog again . . .

Naps, which were starting to become something that may actually be working, are now a no go area. Those babies that were happy to be put down asleep may start to want 'contact naps' again (when they fall asleep physically on you). The usual techniques for getting them off to sleep may stop working. You thought you had their sleep cues/nap patterns figured out, but now they seem like they're tired but fight going to sleep . . . Are they tired or aren't they? They're suddenly sleeping a lot less and they're grouchy, so they must be tired, surely? So you end up spending the day trying to cajole them into sleeping. If you do get them off, it doesn't last long before – 'ping' –their eyes are open.

It's okay. This is all hard, but normal.

Night-time sleep is not much better. Frequent and very frequent night waking rears its ugly head. The first few days you kinda cope okay, because it's like another growth spurt, but when it carries on for longer, you start to get really exhausted. You reach out to a friend/family member/Facebook group and get told something like 'Four month sleep regression – it's a killer', and then get regaled with people's tales of sleep regressions that went on for months and months. There's nothing quite so 'helpful' as hearing: 'We still wake every 40 minutes and she's 33.7 months now!'

It can actually make you feel really quite low, and now that your baby isn't a newborn, people don't have the same sympathy about exhaustion. And well-meaning family members may start telling you to sleep train (don't – it's horrible for all involved and rarely sorts the issue; feeding them back to sleep is the quickest, easiest way and doesn't cause any long term habits or problems). Your neighbour tells you that perhaps the quality of your milk isn't good, and formula or food might help (again, nah, the quality of your milk is just fine, and research shows these things don't make them sleep longer anyway).

You're beyond exhausted now and not finding any solution you feel comfortable with. The woman in the queue at the post office tells you to 'enjoy every moment, it goes so fast', and while you know she's right, you do want to swear at her a bit. Look, it does pass, but, yes, it really can suck and I'm sorry. Call in any favours you're owed, get in laws to cook for you, get a friend to clean for you. Do whatever you can to make life as easy as possible, and that includes at night. This is often the point people start to safely bedshare, for example.

In the evening, you may well have a battle with yourself about how to use that hour where the baby might actually settle . . . do you get some sleep too? Or do you spend some desperately needed me-time? Some of you might have been leaving the baby with your partner and a bottle up to this point, and yet you may find this new unpredictable baby doesn't want a bottle anymore. This can be extremely difficult and make you feel quite resentful at times (I hear you – I was you).

They may also become fussy about which breast they want. My tip is to try feeding them from the less preferred side when they're asleep, if it becomes too difficult.

Essentially, it's a really weird age and the days are very long. They are developing so fast and it's almost too much for them to handle. They want a lot of entertainment and can't really do any of it themselves yet, so the frustration is palpable. It can feel like they're constantly a bit hungry and a bit tired but won't do anything about it. It can also feel like your boobs have lost their magic powers. Why don't they cure everything anymore? Why is the baby fighting and yelling at them? Above all, it can really knock your confidence.

Please know you're not alone, and you are doing brilliantly. This stage is hard, wonderful but hard. You are still everything your baby needs, and more. Just remind yourself that it's a time of rapid growth and development and it takes a lot out of you both, but it's actually a huge leap forward. You're going to get through this stage, just as you have the others. You've absolutely got this.

Are they ready for solid foods?

In the UK, the guidance to start solid foods is from around six months/26-weeks-old onward. This changed from four months in 2001, so well over twenty years ago now. Six months is the recommendation of the World Health Organisation, NHS, and the American Academy of Paediatrics.

But still the message to start solids from four months continues to bang around. It's partly because the regulation of baby food allows the packaging to say it's suitable from four months. This spreads the message that there's no problem starting early, but actually we know from research there's no benefit to starting earlier, and it can increase the risk of infection and tummy problems. So it really is best to wait.

Luckily there are signs of readiness for solid foods, and although that's well past the 'fourth trimester', I'm going to cover them briefly here.

You're looking for your baby:

- Being able to sit well, ideally without much support or unaided.

- Being able to pick things up and bring them to their mouth.

- Loss of the 'tongue thrust reflex', which is the protective reflex to push food back out of their mouth with their tongue if they're not yet ready for it (babies are so flipping clever!).

When all three of the above are present, and they're around the right age, then that will be a good time to start gently introducing some solid foods.

These are some things you might hear are signs they're ready for solids but actually are not!

- Watching you eat

- Waking more at night

- Breastfeeding more frequently

It can be hard to wait until six months sometimes. Your friends may start early, the baby foods say four months plus, and you might even hear that starting solid foods will help your baby sleep (it won't, I'm afraid!), so you can find yourself wondering, why not? Starting solids can be a really exciting time too, and, if I'm honest with myself, I tried to justify reasons why my first baby needed to start solids early, when actually it was *me* that was ready to move on to the next stage. In my experience, no one ever regrets waiting until six months, but they do regret starting early. Please do try to wait. It will be worth it.

I'd also recommend looking into baby-led weaning, which is a way of giving solid foods to your baby that doesn't involve pureeing everything, and works with their abilities to feed themselves. This is a reassuring sign that they're ready to eat, and helps them regulate what they need. It's also great for helping them to explore textures and flavours, and to learn *how* to eat.

Societal expectations

As you come out of the fourth trimester, I'm hopeful that you'll be feeling confident enough in yourself and your abilities as a parent that not a lot will make you question it. However, it can be very hard to keep the faith in yourself when you come up against some of the very bizarre societal expectations at play.

For example, we know that babies need love, closeness, and respectful responsive parenting. We know that babies wake at night. We know that babies need to feed at night. There is no age limit on any of these things. But our culture has a deeply ingrained message that none of this is true.

You may well feel like you're swimming upstream, or going against the grain, and it can be really tough. Now is a great time to remind yourself of why you breastfeed, why you parent in this loving and responsive way, why you respond to your baby at night for the 842nd time . . . And if you haven't already got yourself along to a breastfeeding group, go!! These are people that are going to think and feel a lot more like you do about babies, feeding and parenting. Plus, there's often cake. It's a win-win!

Conclusion

So, the first three months are over! I wonder how it was for you? I'm hopeful that, while you may have hit some bumps in the road, overall you've come out of the fourth trimester feeling relaxed, confident, and in love.

If things have been tough, or they still are, know you're not alone and it will get better. As long as you're parenting with love, respect and kindness you can't go far wrong. You're awesome.

Further Reading

Where do I get help?

If you're having difficulties or worries about feeding your baby, there are lots of places that you can get help.

Support groups. Your local area may have support groups running that you can drop into. You don't need to be having any problems to go; you can use it as a place to meet others, have a cuppa, or just get out of the house for a bit. But if you do have any concerns, they may be able to help you, and will certainly be able to make you feel less alone, and show you where to get the help you need if they can't. There is no charge to attend these groups, although sometimes they'll ask for donations for the tea and coffee fund.

Breastfeeding organisations. There are three wonderful organisations that work with breastfeeding parents in the UK. The Association of Breastfeeding Mothers, La Leche League, and the Breastfeeding Network. They have books, websites full of information, and may run support groups. They may also have helplines available locally. All at no cost to you.

Drugs in Breastmilk Service. The Breastfeeding Network have the most amazing free service that supports parents to find out if the medications they need/take are compatible with breastfeeding and find alternatives if they're not. They have factsheets online about the most commonly used medications and there is no charge for this service, though it's worth noting that as a charity they rely heavily on fundraising.

Midwife/health visitor/GP. You can get breastfeeding support from your midwife and health visitor.

Infant feeding team. Your local NHS Trust may have an infant feeding team that you can get referred to if you're having difficulties that aren't resolving or if you need more than basic support. Your midwife, health visitor or GP can refer you.

IBCLC. Some IBCLC lactation consultants work in private practice. This means you pay a fee to work with them at a time and place that suits you, usually in your own home or via video call. Fees vary, but a one-off consultation will cost between £50 and £100 on average.

('Best money we spent on baby things! She absolutely saved my breastfeeding journey,' as one parent I know put it.) You can find an IBCLC local to you by looking at **lcgb.org/find-an-ibclc/**

Association of Tongue Tie Practitioners. This is a website where you can find information about tongue tie, as well as find a practitioner near you, both via the NHS and privately. Private practitioners sometimes work from a clinic base that you travel to, or some come to your home. **Tongue-tie.org.uk**

National Breastfeeding Helpline. This service has a phone line, an online webchat and is also available via Facebook and Instagram messaging. They're open 9.30am to 9.30pm every day of the year. The services are manned by trained volunteers, peer supporters, breastfeeding counsellors, and IBCLCs. More information at **nationalbreastfeedinghelpline.org.uk**.

Book recommendations

Here are some of my favourite books:

Banks, Shel, *Why Formula Feeding Matters* (London: Pinter & Martin, 2022)

Brown, Amy, *Let's Talk About Feeding Your Baby* (London: Pinter & Martin, 2021)

Brown, Amy, *The Positive Breastfeeding Book* (London: Pinter & Martin, 2018)

Brown, Amy, *Why Breastfeeding Grief and Trauma Matters* (London: Pinter & Martin, 2019)

Evans, Kate, *Food of Love* (Brighton: Myriad Editions, 2008)

Hookway, Lyndsey, *Let's Talk About Your New Family's Sleep* (London: Pinter & Martin, 2020)

Marasco, Lisa, and West, Diana, *Making More Milk* (Maidenhead: McGraw Hill, 2019)

Noble, Robyn, *Breastfeeding Works! Even with Allergies* (Self-Published, 2017)

Oakley, Sarah, *Why Tongue Tie Matters* (London: Pinter & Martin, 2021)

Pickett, Emma, *You've Got It In You* (Market Harborough: Matador, 2016)

Ruddle, Lucy, *Mixed Up* (Amarillo, TX: Praeclarus Press, 2021)

Smyth, Carol, *Why Infant Reflux Matters* (London: Pinter & Martin, 2021)

Stagg, Kathryn, *Breastfeeding Twins and Triplets: A Guide for Professionals and Parents* (London: Jessica Kingsley Publishers, 2023)

Online resources

These are some websites that are incredibly helpful:

abm.me.uk – Association of Breastfeeding Mothers

Breastfeedingnetwork.org.uk – The Breastfeeding Network

Breastfeedingnetwork.org.uk/drugs/factsheets
Breastfeeding network drugs in breastmilk factsheets

https://breastfeeding.support
This website is fantastic! Use it as your breastfeeding 'google'.

www.firststepsnutrition.org
A good resource about starting solids and infant milks

App-network.org
Information and support for puerperal psychosis

Kellymom.com
Another useful site, though American so some slight variations

laleche.org.uk – La Leche League UK

https://www.mind.org.uk/information-support/types-of-mental-health-problems/postnatal-depression-and-perinatal-mental-health/about-maternal-mental-health-problems?
Mental health support

www.breastfeedingaversion.com
Support and information about breastfeeding aversion

D-MER.org
A website for those wanting to learn more about Dysphoric Milk Ejection Reflex

Acknowledgements

It's traditional to write some acknowledgements with a book, and I'm so glad. There are some people I *really* cannot thank enough, and want to acknowledge publicly.

Firstly, to my husband, Ian, who is an unwavering source of love and support. His gentleness and care allows me to continue to learn and thrive in ways I didn't think possible. Also, his practical support in looking after the kids and house while I sat busily typing.

To the inspirational Josie, who has been so incredibly kind by reading and rereading this book to make sure it comes across in the way I hoped. She supports families in a way that I wish I could, and will continue to strive for.

To Phil, who has been a source of information, reassurance, and humour that's pulled me out of deep slumps. I mean it when I say, I genuinely couldn't do any of this without you, my dearest friend.

My mum and my sister, who stand by me unconditionally, even when I throw a temper tantrum about things not going the way I want and are always willing to listen and calm me down. You're wonderful. And also to my dad, who is always there for me if I need him.

And very importantly, to the parents I've supported over all these years. You've taught me so much, and I'm sure will continue to do so.

For the Monday Morning Coffee Crew, thank you for the weekly encouragement, toast-buttering techniques, and most importantly the laughs. You make Mondays a better place to be.

And to those of you who have supported me on social media, helping guide me to see the bigger picture, and understand the emotional aspects of infant feeding so much more, thank you. You have truly helped me figure out who I want to be in my role, and I'm forever grateful.

References

The first few days with your new baby

Bäckhed F, Roswall J, Peng Y, Feng Q, Jia H, Kovatcheva-Datchary P, Li Y, Xia Y, Xie H, Zhong H, Khan MT, Zhang J, Li J, Xiao L, Al-Aama J, Zhang D, Lee YS, Kotowska D, Colding C, Tremaroli V, Yin Y, Bergman S, Xu X, Madsen L, Kristiansen K, Dahlgren J, Wang J. 'Dynamics and Stabilization of the Human Gut Microbiome during the First Year of Life'. *Cell Host Microbe*. 2015 May 13;17(5):690–703. doi: 10.1016/j.chom.2015.04.004. Erratum in: *Cell Host Microbe*. 2015 Jun 10;17(6):852. Jun, Wang [corrected to Wang, Jun].

Crenshaw JT. 'Healthy Birth Practice #6: Keep Mother and Baby Together – It's Best for Mother, Baby, and Breastfeeding'. *J Perinat Educ*. 2014 Fall;23(4):211–7.

Evans A, Marinelli KA, Taylor JS; Academy of Breastfeeding Medicine. 'ABM clinical protocol #2: Guidelines for hospital discharge of the breastfeeding term newborn and mother: "The going home protocol,"' revised 2014. *Breastfeed Med*. 2014 Jan–Feb;9(1):3–8.

Flaherman VJ, Maisels MJ; Academy of Breastfeeding Medicine. 'ABM Clinical Protocol #22: Guidelines for Management of Jaundice in the Breastfeeding Infant 35 Weeks or More of Gestation,' revised 2017. *Breastfeed Med*. 2017 Jun;12(5):250–257.

Hill PD, Aldag JC, Chatterton RT. 'Initiation and Frequency of Pumping and Milk Production in Mothers of Non-Nursing Preterm Infants'. *Journal of Human Lactation*. 2001;17(1):9–13.

Holmes AV, McLeod AY, Bunik M. 'ABM Clinical Protocol #5: Peripartum breastfeeding management for the healthy mother and infant at term', revision 2013. *Breastfeed Med*. 2013 Dec;8(6):469–73.

Kellams A, Harrel C, Omage S, Gregory C, Rosen-Carole C. 'ABM Clinical Protocol #3: Supplementary Feedings in the Healthy Term Breastfed Neonate', revised 2017. *Breastfeed Med*. 2017 May;12:188–198.

Moore ER, Bergman N, Anderson GC, Medley N. 'Early skin-to-skin contact for mothers and their healthy newborn infants'. *Cochrane Database Syst Rev.* 2016 Nov 25;11(11):CD003519.

National Institute for Health and Care Excellence (NICE) Guideline No. 98. 'Jaundice in Newborn Babies under 28 days'. 2010. Accessed July 2023 at https://www.nice.org.uk/guidance/cg98

UNICEF 'Getting Breastfeeding off to a good start', Unicef UK Baby Friendly Initiative education refresher sheet 2. (202) Accessed January 2023 at https://www.unicef.org.uk/babyfriendly/wp-content/uploads/sites/2/2020/04/Unicef-UK-Baby-Friendly-Initiative-education-refresher-sheet-2.pdf

Wambach K, Riordan J. (2016) *Breastfeeding and Human Lactation.* Sudbury, MA: Jones and Bartlett Learning.

Takahashi Y, Tamakoshi K, Matsushima M, Kawabe T. 'Comparison of salivary cortisol, heart rate, and oxygen saturation between early skin-to-skin contact with different initiation and duration times in healthy, full-term infants'. *Early Human Development*, 2011 87(3):151–157.

How to feed your baby!

Colson SD. (2019) *Biological Nurturing: Instinctual Breastfeeding.* Amarillo, TX: Praeclarus Press.

Matthiesen AS, Ransjö-Arvidson AB, Nissen E, Uvnäs-Moberg K. 'Postpartum maternal oxytocin release by newborns: effects of infant hand massage and sucking'. *Birth.* 2001 Mar; 28(1):13–9.

McFadden A, Gavine A, Renfrew MJ, Wade A, Buchanan P, Taylor JL, Veitch E, Rennie AM, Crowther SA, Neiman S, MacGillivray S. 'Support for healthy breastfeeding mothers with healthy term babies'. *Cochrane Database Syst Rev.* 2017 Feb 28;2(2):CD001141.

UNICEF 'Supporting Effective Breastfeeding', Unicef UK Baby Friendly Initiative education refresher sheet 3. Accessed Jan 2023 at https://www.unicef.org.uk/babyfriendly/wp-content/uploads/sites/2/2020/04/Unicef-UK-Baby-Friendly-Initiative-education-refresher-sheet-3.pdf.

Wambach K, & Riordan J. (2016) *Breastfeeding and Human Lactation.* Sudbury, MA: Jones and Bartlett Learning.

Watson Genna C. (2017) *Supporting Sucking Skills in Breastfeeding Infants.* Sudbury, MA: Jones and Bartlett Learning.

How do I know they're getting enough milk?

Evans A, Marinelli KA, Taylor JS; Academy of Breastfeeding Medicine. 'ABM clinical protocol #2: Guidelines for hospital discharge of the breastfeeding term newborn and mother: "The going home protocol,"' revised 2014. *Breastfeed Med.* 2014 Jan–Feb;9(1):3–8.

Galipeau R, Baillot A, Trottier A, Lemire L. 'Effectiveness of interventions on breastfeeding self-efficacy and perceived insufficient milk supply: A systematic review and meta-analysis'. *Matern Child Nutr.* 2018;14:e12607.

Genna C, Barak D. 'Facilitating Autonomous Infant Hand Use During Breastfeeding'. *Clinical Lactation.* 2010;1:15–20.

Holmes AV, McLeod AY, Bunik M. 'ABM Clinical Protocol #5: Peripartum breastfeeding management for the healthy mother and infant at term', revision 2013. *Breastfeed Med.* 2013 Dec;8(6):469–73

Morse JM, Bottorff JL. 'Leaking: A problem of lactation'. *Journal of Nurse-Midwifery,* 1989;34(1):15–20.

Karabulut E, Yalçin SS, Ozdemir-Geyik P, Karaağaoğlu E. 'Effect of pacifier use on exclusive and any breastfeeding: a meta-analysis'. *Turk J Pediatr.* 2009 Jan–Feb;51(1):35–43.

Kellams A, Harrel C, Omage S, Gregory C, Rosen-Carole C. 'ABM Clinical Protocol #3: Supplementary Feedings in the Healthy Term Breastfed Neonate', revised 2017. *Breastfeed Med.* 2017 May;12:188–198.

Landry SH, Smith KE and Swank PR. 'Responsive parenting: establishing early foundations for social, communication, and independent problem-solving skills'. *Dev Psychol.* 2006 Jul;42(4):627–42.

Noonan M. 'Breastfeeding: is my baby getting enough milk?' *British Journal of Midwifery.* 2013;19:2.

Sakalidis VS, Geddes DT. 'Suck-Swallow-Breathe Dynamics in Breastfed Infants'. *Journal of Human Lactation.* 2016;32(2):201–211.

Nipple pain and problems

Mitchell KB, Johnson HM, Rodríguez JM, Eglash A, Scherzinger C, Zakarija-Grkovic I, Widmer Cash K, Berens P, Miller B. 'ABM Clinical Protocol #36: The Mastitis Spectrum', revised 2022. *Breastfeed Med.* 2022 May;17(5):360–376.

Barrett ME, Heller MM, Fullerton Stone H, Murase JE. 'Raynaud Phenomenon of the Nipple in Breastfeeding Mothers: An Underdiagnosed Cause of Nipple Pain'. *Arch Dermatol.* 2012 Dec;17:1–7.

Chow S, Chow R, Popovic M, Lam H, Merrick J, Ventegodt S, Milakovic M, Lam M, Popovic M, Chow E, Popovic J. 'The Use of Nipple Shields: A Review'. *Front Public Health*. 2015 Oct;16(3):236.

Dennis CL, Jackson K, Watson J. 'Interventions for treating painful nipples among breastfeeding women'. *Cochrane Database Syst Rev*. 2014 Dec;15(12): CD007366.

Douglas P. 'Re-thinking lactation-related nipple pain and damage'. *Womens Health* (Lond). 2022 Jan–Dec;18:17455057221087865.

Jackson KT, Dennis CL. 'Lanolin for the treatment of nipple pain in breastfeeding women: a randomized controlled trial'. *Matern Child Nutr*. 2017 Jul;13(3):e12357.

Kent JC, Ashton E, Hardwick CM, Rowan MK, Chia ES, Fairclough KA, Menon LL, Scott C, Mather-McCaw G, Navarro K, Geddes DT. 'Nipple Pain in Breastfeeding Mothers: Incidence, Causes and Treatments'. *Int J Environ Res Public Health*. 2015 Sep 29;12(10).

Lawlor-Smith L, Lawlor-Smith C. 'Vasospasm of the nipple – a manifestation of Raynaud's phenomenon: case reports'. *BMJ*. 1997;314:644.

Li R, Zhang LX, Tian C, Ma LK, Li Y. 'Successful management of a breastfeeding mother with severe eczema of the nipple beginning from puberty: A case report'. *World J Clin Cases*. 2022 Oct 6;10(28):10155–10161.

National Institute for Health Care Excellence (NICE) Clinical Knowledge Summary. 'Scenario: Breastfeeding problems – management'. 2022. Accessed July 2023 at https://cks.nice.org.uk/topics/breastfeeding-problems/management/breastfeeding-problems-management/

Zucca-Matthes G, Urban C, Vallejo A. 'Anatomy of the nipple and breast ducts'. *Gland Surg*. 2016 Feb;5(1):32–6.

Weight gain and milk supply

Becker GE, Smith HA, Cooney F. 'Methods of milk expression for lactating women'. *Cochrane Database Syst Rev*. 2016;9:CD006170.

Ditomasso D. 'Weighing the Facts: A Systematic Review of Expected Patterns of Weight Loss in Full-Term, Breastfed Infants'. *Journal of Human Lactation*. 2015;32:10.1177/0890334415597681.

Foong SC, Tan ML, Foong WC, Marasco LA, Ho JJ, Ong JH. 'Oral galactagogues (natural therapies or drugs) for increasing breast milk production in mothers of non-hospitalised term infants'. *Cochrane Database Syst Rev*. 2020 May;18(5):5.

França, EC, Sousa, CB, Aragão, LC et al. 'Electromyographic analysis of masseter muscle in newborns during suction in breast, bottle or cup feeding'. *BMC Pregnancy Childbirth.* 2014;14:154.

Kent JC, Prime DK, Garbin CP. 'Principles for Maintaining or Increasing Breast Milk Production'. *Journal of Obstetric, Gynecologic & Neonatal Nursing.* 2012;41(1):114–121.

Kellams A, Harrel C, Omage S, Gregory C, Rosen-Carole C. 'ABM Clinical Protocol #3: Supplementary Feedings in the Healthy Term Breastfed Neonate', revised 2017. *Breastfeed Med.* 2017 May;12:188–198.

Marasco L, Marmet C, Shell E. 'Polycystic ovary syndrome: a connection to insufficient milk supply?' *J Hum Lact.* 2000 May;16(2):143–8.

Morton J, Hall J, Wong R et al. 'Combining hand techniques with electric pumping increases milk production in mothers of preterm infants'. *J Perinatol.* 2009;29:757–764.

National Institute for Health Care Excellence (NICE) Clinical Knowledge Summary. 'Scenario: Weight loss in the first few days after birth'. 2018. Accessed July 2023 at https://cks.nice.org.uk/topics/faltering-growth/management/weight-loss-in-the-first-few-days-after-birth/

Neifert MR. 'Prevention of breastfeeding tragedies'. *Pediatr Clin North Am.* 2001 Apr;48(2):273–97.

Neville MC, Keller R, Seacat J, Lutes V, Neifert M, Casey C, Allen J, Archer P. 'Studies in human lactation: milk volumes in lactating women during the onset of lactation and full lactation'. *Am J Clin Nutr.* 1988 Dec;48(6):1375–86.

World Health Organisation. 'Weight for age charts'. Accessed Jan 2023 https://www.who.int/toolkits/child-growth-standards/standards/weight-for-age

World Health Organisation. 'Guideline: Protecting, supporting and promoting Breastfeeding in facilities providing newborn services'. Accessed Jan 2023 at https://apps.who.int/iris/bitstream/handle/10665/259386/9789241550086-eng.pdf

Breast pain and problems

Berens P, Eglash A, Malloy M, Steube AM. 'ABM Clinical Protocol #26: Persistent Pain with Breastfeeding'. *Breastfeed Med.* 2016 Mar;11(2):46–53.

Cotterman KJ. 'Reverse Pressure Softening: A Simple Tool to Prepare Areola for Easier Latching During Engorgement'. *Journal of Human Lactation.* 2004;20(2):227–237.

Joint Formulary Committee (2022). *British national formulary 83*. London: BMJ Publishing and the Royal Pharmaceutical Society.

Kernerman E, Park E. 'Severe Breast Pain Resolved with Pectoral Muscle Massage'. *Journal of Human Lactation*. 2014;30(3):287–291.

Mitchell KB, Johnson HM, Eglash A. 'ABM Clinical Protocol #30: Breast Masses, Breast Complaints, and Diagnostic Breast Imaging in the Lactating Woman'. *Breastfeed Med*. 2019 May;14(4):208–214.

Mitchell KB, Johnson HM, Rodríguez JM, Eglash A, Scherzinger C, Zakarija-Grkovic I, Cash KW, Berens P, Miller B. 'Academy of Breastfeeding Medicine Clinical Protocol #36: The Mastitis Spectrum', revised 2022. *Breastfeed Med*. 2022 May;17(5):360–376.

Expressing

Forster DA, Moorhead AM, Jacobs SE, Davis PG, Walker SP, McEgan KM, Opie GF, Donath SM, Gold L, McNamara C, Aylward A, East C, Ford R, Amir LH. 'Advising women with diabetes in pregnancy to express breastmilk in late pregnancy (Diabetes and Antenatal Milk Expressing [DAME]): a multicentre, unblinded, randomised controlled trial'. *The Lancet*. 2017;389(10085):2204–2213.

Eglash A, Simon L. 'ABM Clinical Protocol #8: Human Milk Storage Information for Home Use for Full-Term Infants', revised 2017. *Breastfeed Med*. 2017 Sep;12(7):390–395. doi: 10.1089/bfm.2017.29047.aje. Epub 2017 Jun 29. Erratum in: *Breastfeed Med*. 2018 Jul/Aug;13(6):459.

Geddes DT, Gridneva Z, Perrella SL, Mitoulas LR, Kent JC, Stinson LF, Lai CT, Sakalidis V, Twigger AJ, Hartmann PE. '25 Years of Research in Human Lactation: From Discovery to Translation'. *Nutrients*. 2021 Aug 31;13(9):3071.

Morton J, Hall J, Wong R et al. 'Combining hand techniques with electric pumping increases milk production in mothers of preterm infants'. *J Perinatol*. 2009;29:757–764.

Neville MC, Keller R, Seacat J, Lutes V, Neifert M, Casey C, Allen J, Archer P. 'Studies in human lactation: milk volumes in lactating women during the onset of lactation and full lactation'. *Am J Clin Nutr*. 1988 Dec;48(6):1375–8.

UNICEF. 'Hand Expressing, Unicef UK Baby Friendly Initiative education refresher sheet 4'. Accessed July 2023 at https://www.unicef.org.uk/babyfriendly/wp-content/uploads/sites/2/2020/04/Unicef-UK-Baby-Friendly-Initiative-education-refresher-sheet-4.pdf

UNICEF. 'Responsive Bottle feeding, Unicef UK Baby Friendly Initiative education refresher sheet 6'. Accessed July 2023 at https://www.unicef.org.uk/babyfriendly/wp-content/uploads/sites/2/2020/04/Unicef-UK-Baby-Friendly-Initiative-education-refresher-sheet-6.pdf

Reflux

Gieruszczak-Białek D, Konarska Z, Skorka A, Vandenplas Y, Szajewska H. 'No Effect of Proton Pump Inhibitors on Crying and Irritability in Infants: Systematic Review of Randomized Controlled Trials'. *J Pediatr*. 2015 Mar;166(3):767–70.

Hassall E. 'Over-prescription of acid-suppressing medications in infants: how it came about, why it's wrong, and what to do about it'. *J Pediatr*. 2012 Feb; 160(2):193–8.

Hegar B, Dewanti NR, Kadim M, Alatas S, Firmansyah A, Vandenplas Y. 'Natural evolution of regurgitation in healthy infants'. *Acta Paediatr*. 2009 Jul;98(7):1189–93.

Hyman P. 'Childhood Defecation Disorders: Constipation and Stool Incontinence'. International Foundation for Gastrointestinal Disorders. Accessed Jan 2023 at 810-Childhood-Defecation-Disorders-Constipation-and-Soiling-1.pdf (iffgd.org).

Joint Formulary Committee. (2022). *British national formulary 83*. London: BMJ Publishing and the Royal Pharmaceutical Society.

National Institute for Health and Care Excellence (NICE). 'Gastro-oesophageal reflux disease in children and young people: diagnosis and management'. Nice Guideline NG1. 2015. Accessed July 2023 at https://www.nice.org.uk/guidance/ng1

Smyth, C (2021) *Why Reflux Matters*. London: Pinter and Martin.

Colic, wind and difficult evenings

Biagioli E, Tarasco V, Lingua C, Moja L, Savino F. 'Pain-relieving agents for infantile colic'. *Cochrane Database Syst Rev*. 2016 Sep 16;9(9):CD009999.

Canivet C, Jakobsson I, Hagander B. 'Colicky infants according to maternal reports in telephone interviews and diaries: a large Scandinavian study'. *J Dev Behav Pediatr*. 2002 Feb;23(1):1–8.

Cohen Engler A, Hadash A, Shehadeh N, Pillar G. 'Breastfeeding may improve nocturnal sleep and reduce infantile colic: potential role of breast milk melatonin'. *Eur J Pediatr*. 2012 Apr;171(4):729–32.

Hill DJ, Roy N, Heine RG, Hosking CS, Francis DE, Brown J, Speirs B, Sadowsky

J, Carlin JB. 'Effect of a low-allergen maternal diet on colic among breastfed infants: a randomized, controlled trial'. *Pediatrics*. 2005 Nov;116(5):e709–15.

Howard CR, Lanphear N, Lanphear BP, Eberly S, Lawrence RA. 'Parental responses to infant crying and colic: the effect on breastfeeding duration'. *Breastfeed Med*. 2006 Autumn;1(3):146–55.

Hunziker UA, Barr RG. 'Increased carrying reduces infant crying: a randomized controlled trial'. *Pediatrics*. 1986 May;77(5):641–8.

Jakobsson I, Lindberg T. 'Cow's milk proteins cause infantile colic in breast-fed infants: a double-blind crossover study'. *Pediatrics*. 1983 Feb;71(2):268–71.

Leung, A; Lemay, I-F, 'Infantile Colic: a review', *J R Soc Promot Health*, 2004 Jul;124(4):162–6.

Lucassen P. 'Colic in infants'. *BMJ Clin Evid*. 2015 Aug;11:0309.

Metcalf TJ, Irons TG, Sher LD, Young PC. 'Simethicone in the treatment of infant colic: a randomized, placebo-controlled, multicenter trial'. *Pediatrics*. 1994 Jul;94(1):29–34.

National Institute for Health Care Excellence (NICE) Clinical Knowledge Summary. 'Scenario: Colic – infantile'. Revised 2022. Accessed July 2023 at https://cks.nice.org.uk/topics/colic-infantile/

Saavedra, MA, et al. 'Infantile colic incidence and associated risk factors: a cohort study'. *J Pediatr* (Rio J). 2003 79(2):115–22.

Wambach, K, & Riordan, J (2016) *Breastfeeding and human lactation*. Sudbury, MA: Jones and Bartlett Learning.

Allergies and the breastfed baby

Academy of Breastfeeding Medicine. 'ABM Clinical Protocol #24: Allergic Proctocolitis in the Exclusively Breastfed Infant'. Breastfeed Med. 2011 Dec;6(6):435-40.

Di Costanzo M, Berni Canani R. 'Lactose Intolerance: Common Misunderstandings'. *Ann Nutr Metab*. 2018;73(suppl 4):30–37.

Fiocchi A, Brozek J, Schünemann H, Bahna SL, von Berg A, Beyer K, Bozzola M, Bradsher J, Compalati E, Ebisawa M, Guzmán MA, Li H, Heine RG, Keith P, Lack G, Landi M, Martelli A, Rancé F, Sampson H, Stein A, Terracciano L, Vieths S. 'World Allergy Organization (WAO) Diagnosis and Rationale for Action against Cow's Milk Allergy (DRACMA) Guidelines'. *Pediatr Allergy Immunol*. 2010 Jul;21 Suppl 21:1–125.

References

Luyt, D. 'BSACI guideline for the diagnosis and management of cow's milk allergy'. *Clinical & Experimental Allergy*. 2014; 44:642–672.

Minchin, M (2015) *Milk Matters: Infant feeding and immune disorder*. Vermont, Australia: BookPOD.

National Institute for Health and Care Excellence (NICE). 'Food allergy in under 19s: assessment and diagnosis'. 2011. Accessed July 2023 at https://www.nice.org.uk/guidance/cg116

NIAID-Sponsored Expert Panel; Boyce JA, Assa'ad A, Burks AW, Jones SM, Sampson HA, Wood RA, Plaut M, Cooper SF, Fenton MJ, Arshad SH, Bahna SL, Beck LA, Byrd-Bredbenner C, Camargo CA Jr, Eichenfield L, Furuta GT, Hanifin JM, Jones C, Kraft M, Levy BD, Lieberman P, Luccioli S, McCall KM, Schneider LC, Simon RA, Simons FE, Teach SJ, Yawn BP, Schwaninger JM. 'Guidelines for the diagnosis and management of food allergy in the United States: report of the NIAID-sponsored expert panel'. *J Allergy Clin Immunol*. 2010 Dec;126(6 Suppl):S1–5.

Tongue tie

de Oliveira AJ, Duarte DA, Diniz MB. 'Oral Anomalies In Newborns: An Observational Cross-Sectional Study'. *J Dent Child (Chic)*. 2019 May 15;86(2):75-80. PMID: 31395111.

Francis, David O., Shanthi Krishnaswami, and Melissa McPheeters. 'Treatment of ankyloglossia and breastfeeding outcomes: a systematic review'. *Pediatrics*. 2015 Jun; 135(6): e1458–e1466.

Hazelbaker, A (2005) *Tongue-tie: Morphogenesis, Impact, Assessment, and Treatment*. Columbus, OH: PanSophia Press.

Hogan M, Westcott C, Griffiths M. 'Randomized, controlled trial of division of tongue-tie in infants with feeding problems'. *J Paediatr Child Health*. 2005 May-Jun;41(5–6):246–50.

LeFort Y, Evans A, Livingstone V, Douglas P, Dahlquist N, Donnelly B, Leeper K, Harley E, Lappin S. 'Academy of Breastfeeding Medicine Position Statement on Ankyloglossia in Breastfeeding Dyads'. *Breastfeed Med*. 2021 Apr;16(4):278–281.

Long T & Finigan, V. 'The effectiveness of frenulotomy on infant feeding outcomes: a systematic review'. *Evidence Based Midwifery*. 2012;11:40–45.

Messner AH, Walsh J, Rosenfeld RM, et al. 'Clinical Consensus Statement: Ankyloglossia in Children'. *Otolaryngology–Head and Neck Surgery*. 2020;162(5):597–611.

National Institute for Health and Care Excellence (NICE). 'Division of ankyloglossia (tongue tie) for breastfeeding'. 2005. Accessed July 2023 at https://www.nice.org.uk/guidance/ipg149

Oakley S (2021) *Why Tongue Tie Matters*. London: Pinter and Martin.

Power RF, Murphy JF. 'Tongue-tie and frenotomy in infants with breastfeeding difficulties: achieving a balance'. *Arch Dis Child*. 2015 May;100(5):489–94.

Segal LM, *et al*. 'Prevalence, diagnosis, and treatment of ankyloglossia: methodologic review'. *Canadian Family Physician*. 2007;53(6):1027–1033.

Watson GC (2016) *Supporting Sucking Skills in Breastfeeding Infants*. Sudbury, MA: Jones and Bartlett Learning.

Myths

Banks, S (2022) *Why Formula Feeding Matters*. London: Pinter and Martin.

Bartick M, Hernández-Aguilar MT, Wight N, Mitchell KB, Simon L, Hanley L, Meltzer-Brody S, Lawrence RM. 'ABM Clinical Protocol #35: Supporting Breastfeeding During Maternal or Child Hospitalization'. *Breastfeed Med*. 2021 Sep;16(9):664–674.

Berens P, Eglash A, Malloy M, Steube AM. 'ABM Clinical Protocol #26: Persistent Pain with Breastfeeding'. *Breastfeed Med*. 2016 Mar;11(2):46–53.

Berens P, Labbok M. 'ABM Clinical Protocol #13: Contraception During Breastfeeding', revised 2015. *Breastfeed Med*. 2015 Jan-Feb;10(1):3–12.

Bergman NJ. 'Neonatal stomach volume and physiology suggest feeding at 1-h intervals'. *Acta Paediatr*. 2013 Aug;102(8):773–7.

Brown A, Arnott B. 'Breastfeeding duration and early parenting behaviour: the importance of an infant-led, responsive style'. *PLoS One*. 2014 Feb;12:9(2).

Canadian Paediatric Society. 'Iron needs of babies and children'. *Paediatr Child Health*. 2007 Apr;12(4):333–6.

deMontigny F, Gervais C, Larivière-Bastien D, St-Arneault K. 'The role of fathers during breastfeeding'. *Midwifery*. 2018;58:6–12.

Doan T, Gay CL, Kennedy HP, Newman J, Lee KA. 'Nighttime breastfeeding behavior is associated with more nocturnal sleep among first-time mothers at one month postpartum'. *J Clin Sleep Med*. 2014 Mar 15;10(3):313–9.

Foong SC, Tan ML, Foong WC, Marasco LA, Ho JJ, Ong JH. 'Oral galactagogues (natural therapies or drugs) for increasing breast milk production in mothers of non-hospitalised term infants'. *Cochrane Database Syst Rev*. 2020 May 18;5(5).

References

Geddes DT, Gridneva Z, Perrella SL, Mitoulas LR, Kent JC, Stinson LF, Lai CT, Sakalidis V, Twigger AJ, Hartmann PE. '25 Years of Research in Human Lactation: From Discovery to Translation'. *Nutrients*. 2021 Aug 31;13(9):3071.

Jeong G, Park SW, Lee YK, Ko SY, Shin SM. 'Maternal food restrictions during breastfeeding'. *Korean J Pediatr*. 2017 Mar;60(3):70-76. doi: 10.3345/kjp.2017. 60.3.70. Epub 2017 Mar 27.

Haastrup MB, Pottegård A, Damkier P. 'Alcohol and breastfeeding'. *Basic Clin Pharmacol Toxicol*. 2014 Feb;114(2):168–73.

Linde K, Lehnig F, Nagl M, Kersting A. 'The association between breastfeeding and attachment: A systematic review'. *Midwifery*. 2020 Feb;81:102592.

Marasco L, West D (2020) *Making More Milk*. Second edition. New York: McGraw Hill.

Liu X, Chen H, An M, Yang W, Wen Y, Cai Z, Wang L, Zhou Q. 'Recommendations for breastfeeding during Coronavirus Disease 2019 (COVID-19) pandemic'. *Int Breastfeed J*. 2022 Apr 11;17(1):28.

Mitoulas LR, *et al*. 'Variation in fat, lactose and protein in human milk over 24h and throughout the first year of lactation'. *Br J Nutr*. 2002 Jul;88(1):29–37.doi: 10.1079/BJNBJN2002579.

Ramsay DT, *et al*. 'Ultrasound imaging of milk ejection in the breast of lactating women'. *Pediatrics*. 2004 Feb;113(2):361–7.

Rinker B, Veneracion M, Walsh CP. 'The effect of breastfeeding on breast aesthetics'. *Aesthet Surg J*. 2008 Sep-Oct;28(5):534–7.

Ruddle L (2021) *Mixed Up*. Amarillo, TX: Praeclarus Press.

Tunc VT, Camurdan AD, Ilhan MN, Sahin F, Beyazova U. 'Factors associated with defecation patterns in 0-24-month-old children'. *Eur J Pediatr*. 2008 Dec;167(12):1357–62.

Vazirinejad R, Darakhshan S, Esmaeili A, Hadadian S. 'The effect of maternal breast variations on neonatal weight gain in the first seven days of life'. *Int Breastfeed J*. 2009 Nov 18;4:13.

Mental health, birth trauma and when things don't work out as planned

Borra C, Iacovou M, Sevilla A. 'New evidence on breastfeeding and postpartum depression: the importance of understanding women's intentions'. *Matern Child Health J*. 2015 Apr;19(4):897–907.

Brown A (2016) *Why Breastfeeding Grief and Trauma Matter*. London: Pinter and Martin.

Chmielewska B, Barratt I, Townsend R, Kalafat E, van der Meulen J, Gurol-Urganci I, O'Brien P, Morris E, Draycott T, Thangaratinam S, Le Doare K, Ladhani S, von Dadelszen P, Magee L, Khalil A. 'Effects of the COVID-19 pandemic on maternal and perinatal outcomes: a systematic review and meta-analysis'. *Lancet Glob Health*. 2021 Jun;9(6):e759-e772. Erratum 052.in: *Lancet Glob Health*. 2021 Jun;9(6):e758.

Collardeau F, Corbyn B, Abramowitz J, Janssen PA, Woody S, Fairbrother N. 'Maternal unwanted and intrusive thoughts of infant-related harm, obsessive-compulsive disorder and depression in the perinatal period: study protocol'. *BMC Psychiatry*. 2019 Mar 21;19(1):94.

Degner D. 'Differentiating between "baby blues", severe depression, and psychosis'. *BMJ*. 2017 Nov 10;359:j4692.

Dennis CL, McQueen K. 'Does maternal postpartum depressive symptomatology influence infant feeding outcomes?' *Acta Paediatr*. 2007 Apr;96(4):590–4.

Fairbrother N, Woody SR. New mothers' thoughts of harm related to the newborn. *Arch Womens Ment Health*. 2008 Jul;11(3):221–9.

Figueiredo B, Dias CC, Brandão S, Canário C, Nunes-Costa R. 'Breastfeeding and postpartum depression: state of the art review'. *J Pediatr* (Rio J). 2013 Jul-Aug;89(4):332–8.

Kendall-Tackett K. 'A new paradigm for depression in new mothers: the central role of inflammation and how breastfeeding and anti-inflammatory treatments protect maternal mental health'. *Int Breastfeed J*. 2007 Mar 30;2:6.

National Institute for Health and Care Excellence (NICE). 'Antenatal and post-natal mental health: Clinical management and service guidance'. 2014 (updated 2020). Accessed July 2023 at https://www.nice.org.uk/guidance/cg192.

Ruddle L (2020) *Relactation*. Amarillo, TX: Praeclarus Press.

Russell EJ, Fawcett JM, Mazmanian D. 'Risk of obsessive-compulsive disorder in pregnant and postpartum women: a meta-analysis'. *J Clin Psychiatry*. 2013 Apr;74(4):377–85.

For partners, friends and family

Baldwin S, Bick D, Spiro A. 'Translating fathers' support for breastfeeding into practice'. *Prim Health Care Res Dev*. 2021 Nov 3;22:e60.

Giugliani ERJ, Caiaffa WT, Vogelhut J, Witter FR, Perman JA. 'Effect of Breastfeeding Support from Different Sources on Mothers' Decisions to Breastfeed'. *Journal of Human Lactation*. 1994;10(3):157–161.

References

Juntereal NA, Spatz DL. 'Breastfeeding experiences of same-sex mothers'. *Birth*. 2020 Mar;47(1):21–28. doi: 10.1111/birt.12470. Epub 2019 Nov 18.

Kong SK, Lee DT. 'Factors influencing decision to breastfeed'. *J Adv Nurs*. 2004 May;46(4):369–79.

Rempel LA, Rempel JK, Moore KCJ. 'Relationships between types of father breastfeeding support and breastfeeding outcomes'. *Matern Child Nutr*. 2017 Jul;13(3):e12337.

Sherriff N, Hall V. 'Engaging and supporting fathers to promote breastfeeding: a new role for Health Visitors?' *Scand J Caring Sci*. 2011 Sep;25(3):467–75.

Coming out of the fourth trimester

Brown A, Harries V. 'Infant sleep and night feeding patterns during later infancy: association with breastfeeding frequency, daytime complementary food intake, and infant weight'. *Breastfeed Med*. 2015 Jun;10(5):246–52.

Douglas PS, Hill PS. 'Behavioral sleep interventions in the first six months of life do not improve outcomes for mothers or infants: a systematic review'. *J Dev Behav Pediatr*. 2013 Sep;34(7):497–507.

First Steps Nutrition Trust. 'Eating well in the first year'. Accessed Jan 2023 at https://static1.squarespace.com/static/59f75004f09ca48694070f3b/t/5a5a41479140b7e31a75ccbc/1515864404727/Eating_well_the_first_year_Sep_17_small.pdf

Kramer MS, Kakuma R. 'Optimal duration of exclusive breastfeeding'. *Cochrane Database Syst Rev*. 2012 Aug 15;2012(8):CD003517.

Landry SH, Smith KE, Swank PR. 'Responsive parenting: establishing early foundations for social, communication, and independent problem-solving skills'. *Dev Psychol*. 2006 Jul;42(4):627–42.

World Health Organization (2001) 'The optimal duration of exclusive breastfeeding'. Report of an Expert Consultation. Accessed July 2023 at https://apps.who.int/iris/bitstream/handle/10665/67219/WHO_NHD_01.09.pdf

World Health Organization (2004) 'The importance of caregiver-child interactions for the survival and healthy development of young children'. Accessed Jan 2023 at https://apps.who.int/iris/bitstream/handle/10665/42878/924159134X.pdf

Index

Index